Becoming Assertive

A Guide for Nurses

Becoming Assertive

A Guide for Nurses

Sonya J. Herman

Johns Hopkins University

D. VAN NOSTRAND COMPANY
New York   Cincinnati   Toronto   London   Melbourne

This book is dedicated to my daughters
Rachel, Marit, and Sarah
for their continuing caring assertions
and encouragements not only to
complete this book but in
everyday living.

D. Van Nostrand Company Regional Offices:
New York   Cincinnati

D. Van Nostrand Company International Offices:
London   Toronto   Melbourne

Copyright © 1978 by Litton Educational Publishing, Inc.
Library of Congress Catalog Card Number: 77-95120

ISBN: 0-442-23259-4

Published by D. Van Nostrand Company
135 West 50th Street, New York, N.Y.   10020

10 9 8 7 6 5 4 3 2

PREFACE

Becoming Assertive: A Guide for Nurses is a self-help book that shows nurses how to apply assertive behavior to their profession. The book is written especially for nursing students, whatever their level of training. It can be used in introductory nursing courses that cover nursing process or interpersonal skills and in care or foundation courses in graduate programs. The book can also be used in a course on psychiatric nursing or community health, trends in nursing, leadership, management, value clarification, program planning, or communication.

Becoming Assertive: A Guide for Nurses is designed to help nursing students improve their communication skills, self-development, and personal and professional effectiveness. Assertive, nonassertive, and aggressive behavior is defined with the help of examples from nursing situations. The book encourages nurses to learn to differentiate among these behaviors and to understand that everyone uses each of them at some time. All of us, however, do not always consciously choose to use or avoid a certain behavior. This book emphasizes the idea that individuals can decide which behavior is comfortable for them in a particular situation. Nurses are encouraged to speak in a self-affirming manner and to express thoughts, feelings, opinions, and beliefs honestly.

The book stresses the interplay of human rights. Nurses are shown how to exercise their rights without denying rights of others. Awareness of one's rights often helps develop self-respect, respect for others, and understanding of the rights of patients and colleagues. Nurses who practice assertive techniques, beliefs, and life styles will more often (1) be authentic personally and professionally with self and others, (2) demonstrate self-direction and self-control in respecting self and others, (3) be more decisive, (4) make a conscious choice in what they think and say to others and how they say it, and (5) be accountable as well as responsible for patient care.

Becoming Assertive: A Guide for Nurses teaches nursing students assertive communication early in their professional lives, enabling them to assert themselves effectively and to intervene in complex interpersonal problems originating in women's sex-role socialization and the traditional nursing socialization process in educational and clinical settings. This book presents assertive training as one way of helping nurses overcome these problems and communicate with patients, physicians, and other nurses in more effective and personally satisfying ways. It gives specific, detailed examples of the many ways in which nurses can use assertive behavior: refuse a request, make a request, ask for a change in behavior, show caring, accept criticism, support patient advocacy and consumer rights. All the examples are based on real hospital or health-care facilities.

ACKNOWLEDGEMENTS

I wish to express my appreciation to all the staff nurses, nurse educators, administrators, supervisors, clinical specialists, nurse practitioners, and students who attended my workshops on Assertion Training, volunteered to fill out questionnaires before, after, and two months following the workshops, and who shared their views of nurses, nursing, and assertiveness.

I owe special thanks to the nursing students in the WRAIN Program who gathered examples of situations involving patients, nurses, and physicians, many of which appear in this book. The Johns Hopkins University Nursing Education Program students, particularly Eunice Bankins, Pamela Norton, and Helen Rogers, contributed patient examples and applications.

My colleague and friend Mary A. Manderino gave me early support in teaching assertive training and permission to use some of her ideas and scripts in this book. I also wish to acknowledge the adaptation of theories of Joseph Wolpe, Arnold Lazarus, and Patricia Jakubowski-Spector, regarding behavior therapy modification, and Albert Ellis, regarding rational emotive therapy.

My research assistant Joan Smith was persistent in coding and keeping track of the research letters and data. My deepest appreciation goes to Mary Hurt, Mrs. Inge Engles, Judy Ingold, and Gloria Lorenzo, who typed and retyped drafts and manuscript.

Sandra Schutz, Mary Manderino, and Merle Paltrow all read the manuscript and gave valuable support as well as suggestions for improvement. My father, Loren Taylor, also read the manuscript and helped me to edit it.

CONTENTS

5. Applying Assertive Behavior: How To Be the Assertive You 78

6. Maintaining Assertive Skills: How To Keep Doing It 113

7. Barriers to Nurses Becoming Assertive: What To Be Aware of and Overcome 122

8. A Look to the Future: Benefits of Assertiveness Training for Nurses   147

Appendix A: Scripts for Assertive Behavior   159

Appendix B: Teaching Nurses Assertive Behavior: Special Considerations   167

Appendix C: A Statement of "Principles for Ethical Practice of Assertive Behavior Training"   172

Index   183

IN THIS CHAPTER:

Students Speak Out
Educators Speak Out
Administrators Speak Out
Nurse Practitioners Speak Out
Nurse Researchers Speak Out

Does Assertiveness Have a Place in Nursing?

Yes, assertiveness has a place in nursing, according to students, educators, administrators, staff nurses, clinicians, nurse practitioners, and nurse researchers. In fact, more than 2,000 nurses taught by this author insist on becoming assertive nurses. These nurses believe in self-respect, respect of others, self-power, authenticity, and in their ability to give competent patient care.

Nurses' interest in learning assertion has occurred for a number of reasons. Professionally, nurses lament the fact that they are disappointed in their choice of careers. Instead of feeling fulfilled and enhanced as persons, many feel they have no control over what they do, that they are not listened to, and, in general, that they are interpersonally exploited.

Because of the extreme anxiety associated with the nursing profession (Menzies, 1955), nurses have had difficulty effectively communicating on interpersonal levels. To counter this nurses have used silence, which has been interpreted as accommodating to the issue. O'Kelly (1976) speaks of nurses as caring persons who believe they must reduce tension and therefore not create any additional tension by reacting in an assertive manner to disagreements and conflict in health settings. Bowman and Culpepper (1974) state that nursing education in the past has occurred in a rigid, regimented, sexually segregated, and often theoretically sterile environment that has not stimulated self-assertion by students but rather passivity and submission to instructors. Upon graduation, nurses are expected to work in hospitals or service institutions within a bureaucratic system in which individuality can be easily overlooked unless the nurse is able to assertively speak up concerning her role in patient care and in the organization. Not being encouraged as a student to speak up for rights on controversial issues to instructors, head nurses, or physicians, the graduate nurse finds that silence has become an established habit.

Not speaking thoughts or feelings in an appropriate manner leads to increased tension and anxiety (Alberti and Emmons, 1974). Continuing this behavior can result in nurses implicitly abdicating their legal right to self-protection or accountability for a patient advocate role. There is ample evidence of nurses' unwillingness to speak up and "rock the boat" in health care institutions (O'Kelly, 1976).

In addition, nurses as a group perceive themselves as powerless (Mauksch and David, 1972; Ashley, 1973; Hall, 1973; Kushner, 1973; Rogers, 1973; Rothberg, 1973). The bureaucracy of the health institutions has often been the excuse nurses have used not to exercise their power and decision-making ability. Bowman and Culpepper (1974) state that nurses in service institutions see people in power as threatening and hostile and, in turn, are not motivated to model after such persons. A closer look reveals that female sex role socialization and the professional nursing socialization of students indicate obedience and nurturing are the acceptable criteria for nurses (Herman, 1977). Further, nurses are taught not to question or challenge (Ehrenreich and English, 1973). As a result, while nurses aspire to have autonomous positions in their dreams, in reality they occupy subordinate positions and give up decision-making powers. Dependent nurse practitioners contrive to exist while allowing other health professionals and organizations to set health standards (Rogers, 1973).

The powerlessness and subservience the above sentences speak to must be reversed for nursing to remain a viable profession—one that is both responsible and accountable to the nurse as well as to the public consumer. Further, nursing research has shown high job turnover rates, and has demonstrated that job dissatisfaction continues to be of concern to hospitals and nurses (Lysaught, 1970; Altman, 1971). This situation is not only a disruptive force in the nursing staff, but contributes to a morale and self-esteem so low that many leave the profession. This behavior is inconsistent with contemporary nursing education and practice, which has a focus of primary care involving a high degree of self-confidence, responsibility, and accountability.

Since the research literature (Lyon and Iranevich, J., 1974; Everly and Falcione, 1976) shows interpersonal relations to be not only an important but primary correlate to job satisfaction for nurses and more rewarding than salary (McCloskey, 1974), it appears extremely pertinent that nurses and the nursing profession learn a way to improve their interpersonal relationships. For these reasons many nurses have found assertive training to be of help.

You may ask how assertive training can particularly help you. Learning assertive responses is a way of decreasing anxiety and helping you begin to develop self-confidence and to trust yourself more. Assertive behavior is one way to help you maintain individuality in a highly technical world; to be accountable for health care to consumers; and to come to terms with the bureaucratic structure of organizations. In addition, the daily use of assertive behavior helps overcome personal frustration and tension encountered in the work life we as nurses encounter.

As you read, you may be thinking this sound great for nurses, but if nurses become assertive, will this help patients? Assertion is self-respect and involves standing up for personal rights and expressing thoughts, feelings, and beliefs in a direct, honest, and appropriate manner without infringing on the rights of others. Therefore, assertion is based on the premise that self-respect cannot exist without respecting others, for example, patients. By respecting your rights, you will more easily be aware of patient or staff rights. Speaking directly to others when your rights are not respected gives them the opportunity to voice their rights or wants to you. At this point, if the views are opposing, negotiation or compromise may take place. Openness to different views helps reduce tension levels and often results in an increase in self-worth for you and the patient, nurse colleague, or physician. When nurses are more direct and sincere, patients often feel freer to voice their concerns more directly.

What do nurses think they will gain from becoming assertive? The following statements were collected from student nurses, educators, nurse administrators, staff nurses, and nurse practitioners in various workshops, discussions, and formal talks.

STUDENTS SPEAK OUT

In the hospital setting, I think that assertiveness would help because I have a tendency to let those who already have their degrees completely overwhelm me with their power, and sometimes I hesitate to speak up when my client is wrong and needs some insight and helpful criticism. When instructors are standing over my shoulder in the clinical setting, I often "freeze up" out of fear that what I say or what I do will be incorrect. Therefore, I believe that if I were more assertive in the hospital setting, I would not be so hesitant and fearful to voice my opinion and try out something new or stand up for my own rights.

Professionally, I can see the value in being assertive as a nurse, having the ability to honestly communicate with a client, and help him or her define needs, wants, and even fears regarding health. Self-confidence and the belief you can help someone are essential to developing a trusting relationship with a client. In working with colleagues it is important to be able to express your beliefs and observations appropriately, yet in a manner firm enough to insure attention.

I feel the need to become more assertive concerning patient contact and relationships with the staff. I want to be able to handle a future position of head nurse with sufficient assertiveness and to be able to direct a patient to obtain optimal care with enough assertiveness as needed.

I need to be more assertive: as a student nurse interacting with patients, in my interactions with my instructors, when faced with any new or unusual situation, and personally in my relationship with my husband.

Assertiveness is self-confidence and self-confidence is something which is essential if you are going to be a nurse. Getting clients or patients to do things which they may not like or appreciate having to do but which are necessary for their health and well-being takes a special knack. I find it hard to tell someone that I feel they are doing something incorrectly, and this situation will be encountered many times in a hospital setting.

Assertiveness is a quality that I have observed in most nurses I look up to. Assertion seems to be necessary for one to survive with the least amount of anxiety and the best communication.

Being able to give more effective evaluations. I need more faith in who I am and how to defend myself when working with more experienced personnel, i.e., staff and instructors so I can feel I do know something and have something to offer. Sometimes I feel very stupid.

Being a student nurse I am sometimes afraid to step out and do what needs to be done, as talking with patients, e.g., being able to ask necessary, but uncomfortable questions or being able to stand up to instructors with new ideas. It's hard not to view instructors as the "parent" figure and their way always being right without question. I have other difficulties, such as: interpersonal relations with teachers, staff and patients; talking in class; talking to strangers, especially patients; getting all the necessary information from my patients for my notes; and most importantly, I took this course because I have difficulty talking and I need to overcome this in order to be an effective nurse. I hope assertiveness will help me in: meeting new people (patients) and being able to talk with them comfortably; not feeling inferior when talking with others, e.g., doctors; expressing my feelings even though they're different from those people I may be talking with; overcoming shyness, embarrassment, and blushing in situations where that shouldn't occur; talking up and asking questions both in and out of the classroom.

I hope that assertiveness in nursing will help me be more comfortable and confident in various clinical situations, as well as everyday life. I feel that if I am more comfortable in giving patient care, my work will be more effective, the patient will be more comfortable and both of us will benefit. I also hope this course will help me in more intimate relationships with the opposite sex, although this is not my primary reason for taking the course. My present major concern is in the clinical setting, especially in dealing with male clients.

EDUCATORS SPEAK OUT

Assertiveness will help me: in dealing with the nursing staff when the inevitable education-service conflicts ensue; to refuse involvement in too many committees; to be a better role model for nurses and patients; and enable me to speak for my rights and patients' rights in inservice education programs.

Learning assertiveness would: enable me to guide students to speak for their rights and enable me to be heard; to be a person; to regain self-respect; to be part of the system—not to be a follower; to be able to do things I would like to do; and not to have to be aggressive.

Assertiveness would help: interactions with people who are in decision-making positions to hopefully arrive at a logical compromise; in working with students to help them learn how to state patient concerns to physician groups; learn how to ask for requests; and learn how to say NO.

I could be a more effective student and patient advocate.

I could be "role model" for students in giving individualized care.

As a clinical nurse practitioner, more self-confidence in me would inspire trust from others. Patients would trust me more and be more likely to follow suggestions.

Assertiveness would help me "know who I am," would put me more in control of my job; gain a positive approach to everyday activities, as working with a department faculty; and help in general, for living in a society where females have been put down.

Learning to assert myself: I would feel more an equal part of the human race; I could help promote change in the health field; and develop better relationships with co-workers.

I think assertiveness would help me develop more self-confidence; thereby become a more effective teacher.

ADMINISTRATORS SPEAK OUT

Assertiveness will help in counseling employees; leadership roles; speaking in group meetings; listening and responding to others.

Assertion might improve my interpersonal relationship skills by helping me be more authoritative in command, but not aggressive; diplomatic; and self-confident. Assertion would stimulate me to pursue higher goals, and to help others to be more assertive by recognizing their weaknesses and strengths.

If I could assert myself, I could better represent the

interests of nursing to hospital administrators and physicians and better communicate with staff, especially in regard to routine disciplinary matters.

I feel assertion would help me limit, in an intelligent manner, my involvement in "extra" activities; be comfortable with myself being assertive vs. aggressive; allow for rational working through of problems/issues; and would free the amount of energy used to deal with internalized feelings for constructive use.

I need to be assertive to assist me in handling situations in which people are hostile, are passive aggressive, and to comfortably discuss and critique policies/problems with administration.

Assertion would help me communicate better with school of nursing administration; help me help students be better change agents; and help staff to be more assertive in behalf of themselves and patients with doctors.

Hopefully to be assertive would help me feel less guilty about having "I need" or "I want" thoughts and feelings and to increase my ability to express my rights and respect others.

Assertiveness would help increase my ability to confront those in "authority" without anger; to increase self-confidence and self-esteem; to be able to say "NO" without guilt; to encourage others to be assertive; and to implement change in a constructive manner without becoming aggressive.

Assertive behavior would help me stand up for my own rights in order to receive recognition due; to recognize and fulfill my own needs in order to decrease my anxiety; and give me more permission to make me happy instead of trying to make others happy always.

Assertive training will help me as an inservice director by establishing me as a role model for other nurses.

I think assertive training will help me feel better about myself, thus I will project a good image.

It will hopefully assist me to achieve a deserved raise.

Assertive behavior may help me to raise the nursing standards of the Bureau of Public Health Nursing.

Client and staff needs will be heard more clearly by administration if nonemotional, assertive communication is utilized.

If nursing is to complete its crisis identity period in health care, systematic assertive behavior is needed.

As a role model for staff, students, and clients, assertiveness would enable me to be open and honest so those I work with would know how I feel and what I think; enable me to clarify what others are saying (be a better listener).

Assertiveness in nursing would enhance setting goals; clarify nurses', mine, and others' rights; and differentiate assertiveness from aggressiveness.

NURSE PRACTITIONERS SPEAK OUT

I feel that the assertiveness training would benefit me in my new role as a nurse practitioner in a setting where I have worked for fifteen years in other roles. I would hope to gain more insight in not only how to be assertive with patients and clients, but also co-workers.

I need an assertiveness training program because one and number one: I do not have any self-confidence and I

am a mousy backward person who can't say NO with
purpose or meaning. People have used me and still do.

I want to change and would appreciate so much help in
learning an effective way of doing so.

I am competent with my practitioner skills, but have a
difficult time convincing physicians and also some
patients.

NURSE RESEARCHERS SPEAK OUT

In 1977 the effect of a workshop, Assertion Training Model
on Anxiety and Assertive Responses of Nurses, was tested. The
Assertion Inventory (Gambrill and Richey, 1975) was adminis-
tered before, after, and two months after in four ten-hour
workshops, in two six-hour workshops, and in a forty-five-hour
course in which the workshop model was taught first, followed
by additional assertive behaviors. The workshop model taught
was similar to the one described in Chapter 4. The 213 nurse
participants were staff nurses, administrators, educators, nurse
practitioners, and clinicians from the East and Midwest who
paid to attend the workshops and who volunteered to participate
in the research project. Student nurses chose to take the forty-
five-hour elective course and volunteered to participate in the
study. Forty nurses who were similar to the experimental group
and were on a waiting list were the control group.
In all workshops the anxiety scores were decreased from pre
to post testing, from pre to two-month follow-up testing, from
post to two-month follow-up testings. The anxiety scores were
decreased at a statistically significant level, and the probability
of using assertive responses was increased at a statistically
significant level pre to post testing in the combined ten-hour
workshops, the combined six-hour workshops, and in the forty-
five-hour course. The control group showed no decrease in
discomfort anxiety scores, no increase in the assertive probability response scores from pre to post testing. Further statistical
results on individual workshops give some support for utilizing a

workshop assertion training model to decrease anxiety and increase assertive responses for nurses—students, educators, administrators, clinicians, and nurse practitioners. Nurses' beliefs were also collected in this research project and are included in Chapter 7.

In another study, Lee (1977) evaluated a cognitive behavioral approach to modifying assertive behavior in hospital-employed registered nurses. A ten-week, twenty-five-hour rational assertion training course was given to seventeen hospital-employed registered nurses. Nine nurses who were on a waiting list were the control group. The experimenter conducted two separate, but similar training classes employing the semistructured group approach as an integrated model utilizing Behavior and Rational-Emotive Therapy (Ellis, 1962). (See Chapter 3.)

Four behavioral tests, including four separate standardized role-playing problematic situations (based on the operational definition of assertion by Lazarus, 1973), and four self-report tests, including (1) The Assertion Inventory, AI (Gambrill and Richey, 1975), (2) The Adult Self-Expression Scale, ASES (Gay, Hollandsworth, and Galassi, 1974), (3) The Wahler Physical Symptoms Inventory, WPSI (Wahler, 1973), and (4) The State-Trait Anxiety Inventory, STAI (Spielberger, Gorsuch, and Lushene, 1970), were given to all subjects at pre and post intervals as a measure of interpersonal communications (self-assertion), levels of anxiety, and the number of physical complaints (symptoms). Compared with the control group, the treatment group of subjects demonstrated a significant increase in assertiveness on the self-report and behavioral tests. There was also a significant decrease in state anxiety and situational discomfort. The training had no significant effect on reported physical symptoms.

Adams (1977) utilized a workshop model on thirty army nurses and used the Assertion Inventory (Gambrill and Richey, 1975) as a pre and post test. His scores pre to post testing showed statistically significant decreases in anxiety and increases in probability assertive response scores.

Other research involving assertion training is being conducted through the School of Nursing Continuing Education Department at the University of West Virginia and in a small study in San Rafael, California.

You now have an idea of how other nurses think assertion would help them, and how it has been used through research. Stop for a minute and consider how it would help you. What do you expect from reading and practicing assertive behavior? Make a list of your expectations and the specific areas in which assertion would help you. It will be useful to refer to this list as you progress toward becoming assertive and through the readings, exercises, and applications in this book come to understand the concepts and benefits of assertive behavior.

REFERENCES

Adams, M. "Assertiveness and Management Training for Nurses." Unpublished manuscript, Behavioral Sciences Division, United States Army, Fort Sam Houston, Texas, 1977.

Alberti, R. E., and Emmons, M. L. *Your Perfect Right: A Guide to Assertive Behavior,* 2nd ed. San Luis Obispo, Calif.: Impact Publishers, 1974.

Altman, S. *Present and Future Supply of Registered Nurses.* Bethesda: National Institutes of Health, 1971.

Ashley, J. A. "This I Believe About Power in Nursing," *Nursing Outlook,* 21 (October 1973): 637–641.

Bowman, R. A., and Culpepper, B. L. "Power: Rx for Change," *American Journal of Nursing,* 6 (June 1974).

Ehrenreich, B., and English, D. *Witches, Midwives, and Nurses: A History of Women Healers.* Old Westbury, N.Y.: The Feminist Press, 1973.

Ellis, A. *Reason and Emotion in Psychotherapy.* New York: Lyle Stuart, 1962.

Everly, G. S., and Falcione, R. L. "Perceived Dimensions of Job Satisfaction for Staff Registered Nurses," *Nursing Research,* 25 (1976): 346–348.

Gambrill, E. D., and Richey, L. A. "An Assertion Inventory for Use in Assessment and Research," *Behavior Therapy*, 6 (1975): 550–556.

Gay, M. L.; Hollandsworth, J. G.; and Galassi, J. P. "An Assertiveness Inventory for Adults," *Journal of Counseling Psychology*, 4 (1975): 340–344.

Hall, C. M. "Who Controls the Nursing Profession: The Role of the Professional Association?" *Nursing Times*, 69 (June 7, 1973): 89–92.

Herman, S. J. "Assertiveness: An Answer to Job Dissatisfaction for Nurses," in R. Alberti (ed.), *Assertiveness: Innovations, Applications, Issues*. San Luis Obispo, Calif.: Impact Publishers, 1977.

————. "Stereotypic Beliefs of Nurses." Paper presented at The Johns Hopkins University Assertion Training Workshop, February 1977.

————. "The Effect of a Group Assertive Training Workshop Model on Anxiety and Assertion of Nurses." (Unpublished research.)

Kushner, Trucia. "The Nursing Profession in Critical Care," *Ms*, 2 (August 1973): 77–102.

Lazarus, A. A. "On Assertive Behavior: A Brief Note," *Behavior Therapy*, 4 (2973).

Lee, C. " A Cognitive/Behavioral Approach to Modifying Assertive Behavior in Hospital Employed Registered Nurses." (Unpublished Master's Thesis.) University of Bridgeport, Bridgeport, Conn., 1977.

Lyon, H., and Iranevich, J. "An Exploratory Investigation of Organizational Climate and Job Satisfaction in a Hospital," *Academy of Management Journal*, 12 (1974): 635–648.

Lysaught, J., *National Commission for the Study of Nursing and Nursing Education: An Abstract for Action.* New York: McGraw-Hill, 1970.

Mauksch, I., and David, M. "Prescription for Survival," *American Journal of Nursing* (December 1972): 2189–2193.

McCloskey, J. "Influence of Rewards and Incentives on Staff Nurse Turnover Rate," *Nursing Research,* 23 (1974): 239–247.

Menzies, I. "A Case-Study in the Functioning of Social Systems as a Defense Against Anxiety," *Human Relations,* 13 (1955): 95–121.

O'Kelly, L. "Revolution in 1976: The Assertive Nurse," *The Weather Vane* (June 1976): 3–5.

Rogers, J. "Theoretical Considerations Involved in the Process of Change," *Nursing Forum,* 12 (1973): 2160–2174.

Rothberg, J. "Choosing to Use Your Professional Prerogatives." Paper Presented to Tennessee Nurses Association Convention, Memphis, Tenn., October 4, 1973.

Spielberger, C. D.; Gorsuch, R. L.; and Lushene, R. E. *STAI manual for the State-Trait Anxiety Inventory ("Self-Evaluation Questionnaire").* Palo Alto, California: Consulting Psychologists Press, 1970.

Wahler, J. *Wahler Physical Symptoms Inventory Manual.* Los Angeles, California: Western Psychological Services, 1973.

Assertiveness: What Does It Mean for You?

Assertion training, while receiving increasing attention in the psychological literature, is also actively gathering impetus on a grass roots level in nursing. Nurses are asking for and attending assertive training workshops for the purpose of improving their communication skills and consequently relationships with clients, physicians, and co-workers. The following brief history and background will give you some insight into the usefulness of being assertive and what assertion is.

BACKGROUND AND HISTORY

The originator of assertive behavior therapy was Andrew Salter, who, in 1949 wrote *Conditioned Reflex Therapy*. He strongly urged developing an assertive personality structure to counteract shyness and avoidance behavior. He stressed specific behavior that stimulates an assertive style of interaction. J. Wolpe, in his *Psychotherapy by Reciprocal Inhibition* in 1958, was the first to identify the term "assertion" in print. He recommended self-assertion for persons who exhibited anxiety and passivity in the presence of others. He believed fears were the reason a person behaves ineffectively with others, and in turn, feels at their mercy. For example, a person who is unable to complain about poor service in a restaurant or hospital usually fears hurting someone's feelings. To explore this further, in 1966 Wolpe and Lazarus worked together to further differentiate the concept of assertion from aggression in role enactment situations. In 1973 Lazarus maintained that the main components of assertive behavior could be classified into four response patterns: (1) the ability to say "no"; (2) the ability to ask for favors or make requests; (3) the ability to express positive and negative feelings; and (4) the ability to initiate, continue, and terminate general conversations. These four response patterns are extremely important and have been the basis for a number of research questionnaire instruments, such as the Behavioral Assertiveness Test (McFall and Marston, 1970) and The Assertion Inventory (Gambrill and Richey, 1975). More important, they have been used as a basis for workshop formats to teach assertion.

Hersen, Eisler, and Miller (1973), who have taught and researched assertion, found that not all individuals behave nonassertively because anxiety inhibits them, but rather because they never learned to assert themselves. This became evident first in the '60s when personal relationships were perceived to be more highly valued and individuals looked to themselves to obtain feelings of satisfaction and self-worth. As individuals adopted different life styles many found that a lack of social skills limited them. Consequently, a sense of personal powerlessness and frustration often existed. John Vasconcellos (1973) speaks of these persons experiencing in the present the most dramatic of all changes: "how the human being views the human being, how man envisions himself as a person, what it means to be human, what consciousness means, what it means to have a body, to express emotions, and to relate authentically." Perceiving personhood and life in an open, positive, and responsible way builds self-esteem. Learning and practicing assertive behavior skills enables individuals to freely and directly express thoughts and feelings to others.

For these reasons many professionals have taught and are teaching assertive training to various populations: college students (Hedquist and Weinhold, 1970; Rathus, 1972; Gambrill, 1973; Manderino, 1974), women (Jakubowski-Spector, 1973; Wolfe and Fodor, 1975), juvenile delinquents (Sarason, 1968), paraprofessionals (Flowers and Golman in press), children (Chittenden, Flowers, and Marston, 1972; Patterson, 1972), and recently nurses (Manderino, 1976; Herman, 1977), in order to encourage active involvement of the individual with others. Thus far, only a few articles in the nursing literature have appeared applying assertiveness to nursing populations (Manderino, 1976; O'Kelly, 1976; Herman, 1976). Educational and continuing education credits are beginning to be given to nurses who partake in such courses and workshops (Herman, 1977).

Perhaps the main reason nursing has been reluctant to support this learning is that the concept of assertiveness has often been misunderstood and confused with aggression. For example, berating the Director of Nursing after being refused a raise or yelling at a doctor because he put you down illustrate belligerence and antagonism—in other words, aggressive behavior. This behavior not only is inappropriate and self-defeating, but it is not compatible with nursing—whose concerns are the nurturance and caring of others. However, the above examples and others that are similar do occur every day in nursing and nurses want to respond in a manner that shows respect for themselves as well as others. Since nurses are very concerned that they not utilize aggressive behavior, the difference between assertive, aggressive, and nonassertive behavior must be carefully clarified.

ASSERTIVE, NONASSERTIVE, AND AGGRESSIVE BEHAVIOR

Assertive behavior is that type of interpersonal behavior which enables an individual to act in his own best interest, to stand up for himself without anxiety, and to exercise his rights without denying the rights of others (Alberti and Emmons, 1974). Assertive behavior is maintaining a balance between aggression and nonassertive behavior.

This balance is maintained by speaking and acting in a positive, direct, and genuine manner. Specifically, assertion is the direct, honest, and appropriate expression of one's thoughts, feelings, opinions, and beliefs without undue anxiety and without infringing on the rights of others. It includes making eye contact with others, smiling, initiating conversations, being able to say "no" in a matter-of-fact manner, making requests of people, and asking someone for a change in behavior. One way it is understood is in relation to inhibited or withdrawn behavior. In the hospital the inhibited or shy nurse may avoid making eye contact with a physician or head nurse when talking, but will instead look out the window or at the floor and lower her voice. The assertive nurse seeks eye contact comfortably, but neither glares nor finds it necessary to stare to overcome any feelings of self-inadequacy. Her voice is firm and sincere. At a restaurant the inhibited person may not return a well-done steak when the order was for a medium-rare steak; however, the assertive individual will mention the dilemma to the waiter and both expect and obtain another steak. In other words, the assertive person is outgoing but not overbearing, spontaneous without being exhibitionistic. If a situation warrants asserting oneself at a later moment because of potential social, financial, or physical sanctions, the assertive person is able to forego immediate gratification.

The assertive nurse is able to say "no" when refusing a request. This occurs honestly and sincerely and as a conscious choice, not because of revenge or angrily getting back at another person. On the other hand, the assertive nurse in the hospital, for example, can ask another nurse to do an extra task or help with another patient because of a genuine need for the request, not to make busy work or because of not liking the other nurse.

Assertion is not continual confrontation, but making a conscious choice about what to say, when, how, and to whom. The assertive professional nurse consciously makes decisions regarding social and work encounters and determines responses pertinent to each situation. In individual interactions some choices are more compatible for her than others. In some situations a decision not to be assertive may be the appropriate choice. For instance, if a patient is dying and the family are anxious, frustrated, or angry with the staff or situation for one reason or another, the assertive nurse can speak to them directly with sensitivity, remain issue-oriented, and will not have a need to retaliate when encountering their frustrations to life's realities. The assertive nurse chooses to remain open to issues, is able to discuss both sides of a conflict, expects others to be assertive, is not a bully, and can compromise as well as win in interactions. While not allowing others to take advantage of her, the assertive nurse does not withdraw, but remains involved in interactions with people. This behavior demonstrates respect for herself and for others involved.

In contrast, the nonassertive nurse hedges when attempting to say "no" so that the other person makes the decisions, even though later this may be resented. Nervousness and anxiety are familiar to the nonassertive nurse as conflict is avoided regardless of the personal cost. Also, she rarely expresses any feelings, but uses avoidance or withdrawal behavior instead. If a disagreement arises, the nonassertive nurse looks at the floor or away from the person involved and feels quite helpless and powerless. In any conflict with nurses or physicians she denies that she has any interpersonal rights. The nonassertive nurse lacks spontaneity, but spends a lot of time talking about others and past conflicts and avoids directly confronting people. Often she feels hurt and sorry for herself and is constantly looking for others, particularly physicians, to rescue or reassure her. This has consequences in terms of patient care; for example, if the unit admits a number of patients and has only one nurse and a technician on the evening shift, the nonassertive nurse may overlook orders, not ask for additional help, feel very helpless and powerless, and spend two hours after work telling anyone who will listen how awful the work situation was. These extremely apologetic people constantly fear they are inconveniencing people and attracting attention. Nurses as well as women in general have been rewarded by society for using nonassertive behavior. Frequently, this is expressed in such comments as "She's so kind, she never says anything but the best about her friends," and "She'll do anything for you."

On the other hand, the aggressive nurse is expressive to the extent that often she dominates, humiliates, deprecates, or embarrasses others by using a loud voice and by not being sensitive to situations. She gives a loud message that she is right and must have her way at all costs. After an encounter with the aggressive nurse others feel devastated and lose self-esteem. The aggressive nurse is often seen as obnoxious or vicious. She obtains what she wants but at the expense of others. The aggressive nurse has to constantly confront others because of internal feelings of insecurity that leave her feeling alienated with only shallow emotional ties. Generally, aggressive people do not go into the profession of nursing or other nurturing professions.

Many nurses use an indirect form of aggressive behavior because of the misery experienced by complete passivity or the resulting isolations from utilizing aggressive behavior. This is the ability to get what one wants by indirect means, such as trickery, seduction, alluding to situations, or manipulations. Society often sanctions this indirectness by implying that women use "womanly wiles" to get what they want. Nurses who express anger indirectly are often the issue in hospitals. The major disadvantages are that the person with whom one is angry may never know if anger is recognized and may never know what the anger is about. Examples of this behavior include the "silent treatment" when one is angry, rather than an assertive "I am angry with you because of," or indirect put-downs ("someone here is sure way off base"), rather than expressing valid criticism directly. A common example is for one nurse to say to others, "Some nurses don't realize the patients don't understand these concepts," rather than suggesting to the nurse teaching the patients, "I think your patient teaching would improve if you would hand out definitions of the concepts you are presenting."

While the above definitions and accompanying descriptions are clear, it is often difficult in nursing practice to recognize the differences between assertive, nonassertive, or aggressive behavior. The following nursing examples will demonstrate these differences: assertive behavior skills such as refusing a request, making a request, asking for a change in behavior, giving and receiving caring assertion, and accepting criticism can be observed in the following examples. The first response is nonassertive, the second is aggressive, and the third is assertive behavior.

WORK SITUATIONS

Assertive Behavior Skill—Refusing a Request

EXAMPLE—WORK OVERLOAD.   Amputee patients require much emotional and physical assistance. You like working with them and appreciate being recognized for your competent work; however, eight patients is unrealistic for one morning's work assignment.

Head Nurse to Staff Nurse: "You work very well with paraplegic patients. I am assigning you to bathe and care for the patients in wards A and B this morning." (Four patients in each ward.)

1. You look down at the floor, sigh, and begin the morning's work.
2. In a tense, high-pitched voice with some giggles, you reply, "You must be kidding," laugh, and make a put-down nonverbal gesture, rolling your eyes to another nurse.
3. In a firm, pleasant voice with a serious look on your face, you reply, "I cannot accept that assignment because four of the patients are so seriously ill they need constant attention. I can take the responsibility for four of the patients, however."

Remarks:

1. If you choose this approach you automatically will be doomed to fail—first with yourself and then your head nurse. On the one hand, you feel flattered that the head nurse realizes you do good work with paraplegic patients, but you realize that in the past you have only been able to care for a few because of the complexity of patient care. Your sigh cannot be interpreted by the head nurse and your nonassertive acceptance of the assignment may end in your feeling depressed or angry at the end of the shift.
2. You can't believe this head nurse has such bad judgment in making patient assignments. It is infuriating to you and you

feel helpless. You indicate this by rolling your eyes at another nurse, hoping for support. She remains quiet.

3. It is obvious to you, based on your experience in this specific patient area, that you cannot handle eight patients. You realize the ward is a little short of help, but that compromising quality of care is not the answer. You clearly assert yourself in stating your limitations and offer to do what is reasonable.

Assertive Behavior Skill—Asking for a Change in Behavior

EXAMPLE—LATENESS. The evening nurse who administers medications has been late to shift report for the preceding three days. This has caused much delay for the evening shift as the charge nurse had to repeat the patient report.

1. In the shift report the charge nurse says to others, "Well, I wonder if Miss X will even show this evening. She's late every day."
2. In a sweet voice, with a smile on her face, the charge nurse says to Miss X, "It must be convenient to make your own time schedule."
3. In a firm, calm voice the charge nurse says, "You have been coming in fifteen to twenty minutes late this week. I am frustrated as I have to repeat patient report and many patients are asking for their medications. I would like you to be on time."

Remarks

1. If you tell others, this is only a waste of time as far as resolving the issue. The lateness can only be corrected by the person exhibiting this behavior.
2. By masking your irritation with a sweet voice and smile, a clear message is avoided and again the issue is avoided, but hostility may be felt.
3. By describing the behavior, the charge nurse directly states her feelings and thoughts about the lateness. This allows

the other person to say what he or she is thinking.

Assertive Behavior Skill—Accepting Criticism and Asking for More Information

EXAMPLE—UNCLEAR WORK ORDERS INVOLVING PATIENT CARE. You do not understand the order for a medication as written so you page the physician who wrote the order. He does not respond for forty-five minutes and when he does come he yells, "What's the matter with you? Why are you looking for me?"

1. You look at the chart in your hands and in a low, shaky voice say, "This order seems, uh, uh, seems not clear" (wishing all the time you had not called him).
2. You snappily respond, "Who are we supposed to look for when an order is wacky?"
3. In a firm voice, with no smile, you say, "I don't like to be yelled at. I was looking for you as I do not find this order clear. Do you want the medicine given in the morning and evening, in divided doses, or just in the morning?"

Remarks

1. You look down and are afraid he will again yell at you. The fact that he raised his voice and sees you avoid the issue may give him permission to do so.
2. You are angry that he yelled at you and return similar behavior to him. Your anger causes you to forget to verbalize that the problem arose from the confusing order.
3. In a self-confident manner you let him know your feeling when yelled at. Also, you specifically mention what is unclear in regard to the medicine order.

In these examples, the assertive response was a basic assertion. In each of the above examples the nurse made a simple, direct reply and stood up for her personal rights, beliefs, and feelings. A more complicated response would include empathy. Many assertion examples in nursing would be of this kind, which conveys sensitivity and understanding to the other person. The first part of the assertive response tells the other that you are aware of or recognize his or her situation. The second part of the assertive response conveys the speaker's thoughts, feelings, beliefs, based on his or her rights.

An empathetic assertion might begin with, "I understand what you are saying . . . but," or "It does sound difficult to do . . . however," or "You certainly are upset about . . . however." Look for this in the first part of the assertive response in the following example.

Assertive Behavior Skill—Giving and Receiving Caring Assertions

EXAMPLE—DEALING WITH PAIN AND SETTING HELPFUL LIMITS. Miss F. (patient) is suffering from painful metastatic cancer. In order to control the pain, she was given a large amount of narcotic medication and has become addicted. Since she is not in the last stage of illness, the physician, patient, and nurse discuss the situation and together decided to alleviate the narcotic to relieve periods of depression with the hope that the patient will be able to resume some of her previous activities despite some painful intervals. The nurse is to help the patient tolerate and deal with the pain to implement this plan agreed upon by patient, physician, and nurse.

Patient (*screaming*): "Nurse, I have tolerated this pain all morning and I can't any longer; do something."

1. In a tense voice you say, "Well, it will get better. I'll go get you some juice, then we'll talk about something else."
2. In a brisk voice you reply, "You agreed to the plan of helping cut out the narcotic; didn't you mean it? You know it will require self-discipline and time."
3. In a calm voice you say, "I understand how difficult it must be to tolerate the intensity of your pain (empathetic assertion)—let's explore some of your thoughts preceding it, as this may help you to cope with it. When did it begin this morning? What were you thinking about this morning when it began?"

Remarks

1. You feel upset and uncomfortable to see that the patient is in pain. As a nurse you want to relieve her pain medically immediately, as it increases your feelings of helplessness. You agreed to the plan but now feel anxious so you offer juice instead, avoid the pain issue, and walk away.

2. By reacting and putting all the responsibility on the patient and adding, "didn't you mean it?" you inflict the additional stress of guilt on a person who is already dealing with the stress of pain. Furthermore, the patient remains unaware that you realize the difficult situation and, in fact, may feel worse, as you offer no sympathy. Instead you return your frustration, which may increase the patient's.

3. In a calm voice you use an emphatic assertion that you hope will help the patient realize you are able to understand this very difficult situation she faces. You will also talk about it more and be assertively involved in helping the patient deal with the pain (Herman, 1977). The following conversation then proceeds:

Nurse *(calm voice):* "I understand how difficult it must be to tolerate the intensity of your pain. Let's find out about the pain, as this will help you cope with it. When did it begin this morning?"

Patient *(tense):* "Oh, I don't know—how can you be so heartless to want to do nothing but talk?"

Nurse: "It may sound heartless, but this is one way of helping relieve the pain. By pinpointing when it occurs we can then look to see what circumstances provoked it. Now, when did it start?"

Patient *(calm):* "Right after breakfast—when I used to get my shot of narcotic."

Nurse: "What were your thoughts preceding the pain?"*

*From "Assertiveness: An Answer to Job Dissatisfaction for Nurses," by Sonya Herman. Edited by R. Alberti, in *Assertiveness: Innovations, Applications, Issues.* Copyright © 1977. Reprinted by permission of the publisher, Impact Publishers, Inc., San Luis Obispo, California, 93406.

In each of the assertive examples you have seen, the response made was based on the interpersonal rights of the nurse involved. For example, the right to know one's own limitations in giving care to others, the right to express irritation and annoyance when another nurse is late and violates your personal right of leaving work on time, the right to make a request to understand more clearly a medical order, and the right to give authentic caring assertion in the example where the nurse helps the patient cope with pain. Each resulted in the individual nurse getting her needs and preferences respected, while presenting the assertion in a way that maximized the likelihood that the other person could assertively respond. Since the purpose of using assertive behavior is to promote honesty and sincerity in interactions with others, you may not always achieve "your" objective. It is neither winning nor losing that is the goal in assertion, but rather emotional honesty in a more equalized interaction in which personal rights and the rights of others are respected.

INTERPERSONAL RIGHTS

Interpersonal rights are intricately connected with assertion. Nurses who believe they have basic human rights more readily give themselves permission to believe and behave assertively. Nurses who believe they have a right to be listened to will more readily insist on saying what they think than nurses who are not aware of their rights. Similarly, nurses who believe they have a right to be respected usually obtain respect from others. Assertive behavior becomes more spontaneous for nurses who can identify their interpersonal rights and the rights of others. In fact, it is necessary to accept and integrate human rights to help overcome the helplessness or powerlessness nurses feel at frustrations encountered while working in the total health care system.

Since learning to be more assertive is the goal for nurses, identifying and believing in human rights is an important first step. Here is a list of basic human rights nurses have found essential:

Nurses' Bill of Rights

The right to be respected—to be listened to.
The right to have and state thoughts, feelings, and opinions.
The right to question or challenge.
The right to understand and have in writing what is expected at work.
The right to say "no."
The right to be an equal member of the health team.
The right to ask for changes in the system.
The right to a reasonable work load.
The right to make a mistake.
The right to make decisions regarding health or nursing care.
The right to do health teaching.
The right to choose not to assert oneself.
The right to be a patient advocate or to teach patients to speak for themselves.
The right to change one's mind.

What additional rights do you choose? Think when you last stood up for a human right in which you believed. Does this happen frequently? If not, why not?

How Do These Rights Get Overlooked?

In the health care system, even though each person has the same interpersonal rights as the next person, outside of work roles and credentials, nurses still tend to evaluate persons in their thoughts on scales in which some are "better" than others. (Refer to theory in Chapter 3 and data in Chapter 7.) Alberti and Emmons (1974) speak to this in regard to the total population— doctors are thought of as better than plumbers, men better than women, whites better than blacks, adults better than children. In the nursing profession, the following is often perceived: physicians are better than nurses, head nurses better than staff nurses, supervisors better than head nurses, and nurses better than patients. Thinking and then acting as if some people have more or less value, and therefore are more qualified to have human rights than others, is not only unrealistic and irrational but may imply to some that neither nurses nor patients have rights. This is an example of how irrational thoughts and beliefs can be responsible for persons ignoring their personal rights. (Irrational versus rational beliefs are explained more in Chapter 3.) The "elitism" of the medical profession has perpetuated some of this irrationality by insisting that physicians are the only people with health information, that physicians must tell nurses and patients what to do, that physicians shoulder all the responsibility for health care, and that physicians have special rights as people because of their work roles and credentials. If irrational beliefs as stated go unchallenged, human rights often are overlooked.

What Happens to Us When We Overlook Rights?

As nurses you do have the same interpersonal rights as others. If you do not exercise these rights, others, such as physicians, patients, and nurse colleagues, will not respect you.

When we deny or ignore our personal human rights this increases feelings of helplessness and powerlessness and reinforces our own nonassertive behavior. This behavior has occurred in nursing not only because of the traditional female sex role socialization process and the educational socialization process of nurses, but because of the extreme literal interpretation of nurses as patient advocates. Historically, nurses have not only demanded food, clothing, and bedding for patients, but have been instrumental in helping patients to express their wants and rights to doctors, other staff, and family members. In fact, because we are so indoctrinated to give to and care for others (patients and staff), many times nurses and others forget they are people who have needs, wants, and personal rights themselves. Equality in relationships has automatically taken second place to patient care for many nurses. In other words, the nursing profession and the individual nurse have not demanded for themselves the same respect they give patients or staff. This does not improve when nurses keep themselves, or are kept, so busy taking care of patients that a habit of ignoring one's own rights becomes established. In fact, this leads to further isolation from thoughts, feelings, opinions, and beliefs, and reinforces a dependency role that lowers self-esteem and encourages nonassertive behavior.

Nurses who do not identify and accept human rights continue to practice nonassertive behavior. They avoid possible conflict, anger, rejection, and do not accept responsibility for feelings. One nurse explained: "I hate myself for not speaking at the meeting on that issue, but at least things remained on an even keel. Besides, our director of nursing always compliments us for accepting solutions and going along with situations and that makes it more difficult to break through and express real feelings." It's clear this nurse has not chosen the right to express her honest thoughts. In addition, the director of nursing is rewarding nurses who accept solutions and situations whether they actually want them or not. If you are dependent on compliments from others, this will encourage the "I hate myself" tensions and avoidance of honest feelings or thoughts regarding the issue being discussed.

Risks, Responsibilities, Consequences, and Interpersonal Rights

Utilizing assertive communication skills entails some personal risks and always involves responsibilities and consequences. When first learning assertiveness it is often more beneficial to work on new behaviors in "low risk relationships" so that you will experience success. Although this differs for individuals, it usually means with those persons who are not intimately or closely involved with you, such as an acquaintance, someone you work with occasionally or with whom you are pretty much uninvolved emotionally.

In the previous example in which the nurse did not risk expressing a different opinion, the consequences would probably be not getting a compliment or approval or perhaps even that the group members would disagree with her ideas. Since this would be a new behavior, she might experience some uneasy feelings herself. However, by asserting herself she might gain self-confidence and reduce tensions incurred by avoiding the situation. The nurse might also learn by speaking, instead of remaining silent, that nothing awful or catastrophic would happen to her. Using assertive communication skills to express your rights helps enhance yourself but also lets others know more about you and see that you are responsible for what you say. This gives others the choice to interact honestly with you by either agreeing or disagreeing. Permission to be yourself and express yourself sincerely to others is the result of claiming personal rights. This permission to be oneself is not to be interpreted as a right to abuse others, but rather by owning personal rights one becomes responsible for personal behavior and the consequences.

Let's look at an example of consequences when nurses exercise their Bill of Rights. One of the rights nurses have chosen is the right to make mistakes—not to be perfect. In choosing this right nurses are admitting their humanness and recognizing that all people sometimes make mistakes. This right does not mean that nurses may make mistakes purposely or be irresponsible and repeat mistakes. Rather, it implies that if mistakes are made, nurses will responsibly admit to them and at the same time learn from them and not repeat similar behavior if at all possible. It means that nurses will not talk themselves out of the right to make mistakes if they make one. For example, giving a wrong medication can be disastrous and doesn't happen often. If it occurs, the nurse need not deprecate herself by thoughts like, "I'm stupid and no good to have made that mistake." "I can't be trusted ever again to give medicines," "No patient is going to want me to take care of him since I made this mistake." Instead, the nurse would strive to maintain assertive rational thoughts, such as "I made a mistake giving that drug to the wrong patient. What can I do now to rectify the mistake?" "I never do that, as I'm always very careful to check the medicine with the patient. Since it happened I'll actively begin to concentrate more on double-checking the medicine cards and the patient. In this way I'll prevent future mistakes."

This example demonstrates the interplay of rational assertive thinking, assertive behavior, and basic human rights plus risks, responsibilities, and consequences accompanying assertion. You will notice that this interplay will be expanded upon as you read further.

REFERENCES

Alberti, R.E., and Emmons, M.L. *Your Perfect Right: A Guide to Assertive Behavior,* 2nd ed. San Luis Obispo, Calif.: Impact Publishers, 1974.

Chittenden, G.E. "An Experimental Study in Measuring and Modifying Assertive Behavior in Young Children," *Monographs of the Society for Research in Child Development,* VIII, Serial #31.

Ellis, A., and Harper, R.A. *A New Guide to Rational Living.* North Hollywood, Calif.: Wishire Book Co., 1976.

Flowers, J.K., and Marston, A.R. "Modification of Low Self-Confidence in Elementary School Children," *Journal of Educational Research,* 66 (1972): 30–34.

Flowers, J.V., and Goldman, R.D. "Assertion Training for Mental Health Paraprofessionals," *Journal of Counseling Psychology,* (in press).

Gambrill, E.D. "A Behavioral Program for Increasing Social Interaction." Paper presented at Seventh Annual Meeting of the Association for the Advancement of Behavioral Therapy, 1973.

Gambrill, E.D., and Richey, C.A. "An Assertion Inventory for Use in Assessment and Research," *Behavior Therapy,* 6 (1975): 550–561.

Hedquist, F.J., and Weinhold, B.K. "Behavioral Group Counseling with Socially Anxious and Unassertive College Students," *Journal of Counseling Psychology,* 17 (1970): 237–242.

Herman, S.J. "Assertiveness: An Answer to Job Dissatisfaction for Nurses," in R. Alberti (ed.), *Assertiveness: Innovations,*

Applications, Issues. San Luis Obispo, Calif.: Impact Publishers, 1977.

―――. "Assertiveness Training," *The Hopkins Nurse,* Issue 4, January 1976.

―――. "The Effects of a Group Assertion Training Workshop Model on Anxiety and Assertion of Nurses." (Unpublished research.)

Hersen, M.; Eisler, R.M.; and Miller, P.M. "Development of Assertive Responses: Clinical, Measurement and Research Considerations," *Behavior Research and Therapy,* 2 (1973): 505−521.

Jakubowski-Spector, P. "Facilitating the Growth of Women Through Assertive Training," *The Counseling Psychologist,* 4 (1973): 75−86.

Lazarus, A.A. "Assertion Behavior: A Brief Note," *Behavioral Therapy,* 4 (1973): 697−699.

McFall, R.M., and Marston, A.R. "An Experimental Investigation of Behavior Rehearsal in Assertiveness Training," *Journal of Abnormal Psychology,* 76 (1970): 295−303.

Manderino, M.A. "Comments on Teaching Nurses Assertiveness," *Journal of Continuing Education of Nurses,* (March−April 1976): 80−81.

O'Kelly, L. "Revolutions in 1976: The Assertive Nurse," *The Weather Vane,* (June 1976): 3−5.

Patterson, R.L. "Time Out and Assertive Training for a Dependent Child," *Behavior Therapy Journal,* 3 (1972): 466−468.

Rathus, R.A. "An Experimental Investigation of Assertive Training in a Group Setting," *Journal of Behavior Therapy and Experimental Psychiatry,* 3 (1972): 81−86.

Salter, A. *Conditioned Reflex Therapy*. New York: Farrar, Straus & Giroux, 1949; Capricorn Books Edition, 1961.

Sarason, I. "Verbal Learning, Modeling, and Juvenile Delinquency," *American Psychologist*, 23 (1968): 254–266.

Vasconcellos, J. Foreward to *Your Perfect Right: A Guide to Assertive Behavior,* by R. Alberti and M. Emmons. San Luis Obispo, Calif.: Impact Publishers, 1974.

Wolfe, J., and Fodor, I. "A Cognitive Behavior Approach to Assertiveness Problems in Women," *The Counseling Psychologist,* 1975.

Wolpe, J. *The Practice of Behavior Therapy*. New York: Pergamon Press, 1969.

Wolpe, J. *Psychotherapy by Reciprocal Inhibition*. Stanford: Stanford University Press, 1958.

Wolpe, J., and Lazarus, A.A. *Behavior Therapy Techniques*. New York: Pergamon Press, 1966 (Now out of print).

3 Assertive Communication Skills

It is helpful when becoming assertive to build a repertoire of assertive verbal and nonverbal communication skills. By learning a number of ways to respond to situations you will develop a fuller integration of thinking, feeling, and behaving as your own personal assertive style grows. You will also notice that these skills can be used alone, but as you become more proficient in combining the skills, it becomes easier to convey greater empathy and sensitivity, or to effect a change in another person's behavior toward you.

VERBAL SKILLS

Think and Talk About Yourself Positively

Actively thinking positive thoughts and making positive self-statements in conversations will not only increase your self-respect, but will also enhance self-confidence and help you begin to build and maintain assertive behavior skills. Otto (1965) found that more people focus on negative thoughts or make statements regarding their problems rather than thinking and talking of their positive aspects. When the majority of thoughts and statements made are positive, the results are greater self-esteem and respect from others. This reduces one's need for approval from others and frees an individual to make decisions spontaneously and handle conflicts directly. In this way one's needs are met and self-control is established. This assertive behavior skill is especially important for nurses who have long been better advocates for patients' rights than for their own. One nurse began this process by thinking in the following manner.

I am an excellent medical nurse. I know the composition and effects of different medicines and which are pertinent for which illnesses. I have good observation and nursing care skills which I utilize each day. I am also able to communicate with my patients and enjoy talking with and caring for them. There are days when I am tired or down, but I actively try to examine any thoughts accompanying those feelings. I share the positive aspects of myself with others, not in a bragging manner, but as seems appropriate. This reinforces me to accept my assertive self and builds my self-respect. Although this was difficult at first, after some practice it comes easier and now I find I'm most interested in sharing those aspects of myself with others and encouraging them to do the same. The increased sense of personal freedom I have discovered is very liberating and stimulates other kinds of personal growth in me. I have found alternatives and choices that formerly I didn't think existed. I began by reinforcing myself by spending 20 minutes doing what I wanted after saying something positive about myself in a conversation. I increased the reinforcer time to an hour on weekends. I also began to think of things I like to do, make a list, and actually share them with others. One time I counted self-statements I made in one day. About this time I found myself beginning to compliment more freely and offer frequent backrubs in the middle of the day. This gain in self-respect was accompanied by increased ability to give to patients and others.

As you read about other assertive communication skills it will be helpful to reflect on this nurse's experience with positive thoughts and self-statements and decide if her learning could benefit you.

"I" Statements

Using "I" statements indicates to another that you are taking responsibility for what you say and feel. Further, "I" statements indicate that you believe and trust your thoughts and feelings and have decided they are worthwhile to share with others. You are able to risk being an authentic person and do not need to blame others. As a head nurse making a statement, you might say, "I do not want Miss Smith to have a complete bath. She is very tired and I think she needs rest." This statement clearly says the head nurse is responsible for the decision not to give Miss Smith a complete bed bath. Using content such as, "You will tire Miss Smith if you give her a bath—you know she needs her rest" only confuses others because of the "you" messages.

Initiating Conversations

Initiating conversations is a most important assertion skill for professional nurses to utilize with patients. Because it sounds simple, it is often not done well, nor is it often evaluated as students work with patients. For example, when you go into a patient's room it is helpful to you and the patient to say who you are (name and your profession) and explain what you would like to do with or for the patient before you do it. The following might occur: "I am Miss Jones, your nurse. I will give you a morning bath and your medications in about fifteen minutes." In this way the patient can respond to you without having to guess what's going to happen, in contrast with Miss Jones walking into the patient's room saying "Hi" in a cheery voice, looking around the room, bringing in bed linen, some ice, and then disappearing for an hour. When nothing more than "Hi" is verbalized, the patient as well as the nurse is prevented from becoming involved in any nursing care given.

Giving and Getting Information

After you initiate an interaction with a patient there are several ways to maintain the conversation, depending on the purpose. If you need to obtain more specific facts in regard to the patient's health, you can make open-ended statements and then focus on detail. For example: Nurse: "I understand from the morning report that you have been uncomfortable during the night with pain." Patient: "Yes, I hurt all over and want some relief." Nurse: "Where exactly is the pain?" Patient: "It's here on the left side of my stomach." Nurse: "Let's look closer," (palpating patient's abdomen). "Does it hurt here? Is it a sharp or dull ache?" etc. Active listening and empathetic responses play an important role in expanding conversations.

When miscommunication occurs, these skills are useful in clarifying issues. For example, you might say, "Did you mean this . . . ." or "I'm not sure I understood—did you ask for . . . ."

Self-Disclosing

Self-disclosing means stating and sharing your own thoughts and feelings with others. It is a method of giving information to others about yourself. For example, if you've found this to be true, you might self-disclose to a patient, "It is painful to have gas in your abdomen and not obtain relief," or "After abdominal surgery you do have a sore abdomen and it is difficult to turn over in bed or get up," or "I was a patient in the hospital last year and I was particularly disturbed when my bell light was not answered immediately" (in reply to a patient complaining about waiting). The follow-up statement might be, "I will look for your light and will return in five minutes." Self-disclosing and clarifying your expected behavior can reduce anxiety in a tense patient.

Giving Constructive Criticism

Constructive criticism is a skill used often in nursing by head

nurses, supervisors, or administrators evaluating others' performance at work. Educators use this skill often in teaching
students. When giving constructive criticism it is important to
begin with an "I" message so it is clear to the recipient that you
are taking responsibility for making the criticism. For example,
"I get irritated when you come late to the shift," or "I think your
uniforms are too short; I would prefer that you wear a longer
uniform," or "I become annoyed when you take a coffee break at
the time the other nurse is off the floor," or "I become annoyed
when I come to the ward and see all the nurses visiting in the
nurse's station." These constructive statements given in a
direct, matter-of-fact but firm tone of voice and an "I" message
allows others to hear them and respond directly with their
thoughts and feelings.

In addition, it may be appropriate to balance both positive and
negative thoughts and feelings when giving criticism. For
example, "Although you give quality nursing care to the patients, I get irritated when you arrive late for your shift." Or "I
admire the way in which you handled the emergency admissions yesterday; however, I found myself getting annoyed with
the short uniforms you wore, as all the patients could see the
tops of your hose when you bent over." Or "I notice, Ms. Smith,
that you give excellent care to the patients. I particularly find
your tone of voice when you speak to them is most appropriate,
empathetic, and helpful. The patients seem quite relaxed after
you have given them morning care. I would like to ask you to
relate more in this way to staff and come on time to work. This
has become a major issue on the burn unit." Balancing positive
and negative statements is a way of saying I care about you, but
want you to think about another behavior which bothers me.

Accepting Criticism

Accepting criticism is an important skill for nurses. Whenever
people work together there is bound to be conflict. Being direct
with one another has the potential to improve the relationship.
One way of dealing with conflict is to listen to the other person's
point of view. If this involves his giving you criticism that is valid

and true, it is important for you to acknowledge the fact. For example, "You are correct, I have been late recently," or "Yes, that one uniform is too short; I've been meaning to throw it out, but when the others are dirty I wear it," or "Yes, I have been taking coffee breaks in the mornings at 10:00 to meet my friends and sometimes the other nurse isn't there."

On the other hand, if the criticism is not true from your perspective, it is still important for you to acknowledge the criticism, but then state your beliefs. For example, "You are correct, I have come late to work recently; however, I worked overtime all last week and the arrangement I made with the head nurse was that I start work thirty minutes later to make up for the overtime I put in."

Giving Personal Criticism

It is much more acceptable to give criticism immediately, simply, and matter-of-factly. How many of us have not noticed small things about ourselves until later when other people did not have the "guts" to tell us immediately. For instance, "Did you realize your lipstick is not straight," or "Tom, it looks like you have some egg in your beard," or "Ms. Smith, your breath smells bad today; why not try this mouth wash." Giving personal criticism these ways are more acceptable than to say, "Ms. Smith, I want to talk to you; now please don't take this wrong, I'm only trying to help you, but it seems like you might want to brush your teeth again. I mean your breath has an odor. Nothing personal, but you might use some mouth wash." It shows caring when we interact directly.

Making Statements Without Explanations

Directly asking others or refusing to do things without apologies or explanations is another assertive skill. For example, "I want you to take Miss Smith and Miss Black their sleeping medications," rather than "Miss Smith and Miss Black are having a hard time sleeping," or saying directly to patients, "No, you cannot drink fluids as yet. I will let you know when."

Persistence

Sticking to the issues at hand in a firm manner often brings positive results. For example, Nurse: "I want a new pain medication order, Dr. Taylor. Miss White was in pain last evening and all night the Darvon compound was given but did not help her discomfort." Dr.: "Well, try two Darvons then." Nurse: "Miss White has taken two and also had a back massage and still is in discomfort. I want a new pain medication order for her." Dr.: "Darvon helps the kind of pain she is having." Nurse: "That may be true, but it has not helped her. She told me she has taken Demerol and obtained some relief. Would you write an order for that?" Dr.: "Oh, all right."

Giving and Receiving Compliments

Giving others direct and spontaneous positive messages is a marvelous assertive habit. Many times positive messages go unsaid. In hospital environments laden with anxiety, stating and sharing honestly what is good or nice about a patient or staff member often uplifts both the other person and yourself. Being able to receive a compliment directly is another skill. Patients often say to nurses, "Thank you so much for answering my light and helping me." An assertive reply of "You're very welcome" or "I enjoy being able to help you" indicates your acceptance, whereas, "Oh, it's my job" or "It's nothing" degrades the original comment. Further, it does reinforce compliments to be given in the future.

Expressing Negative Feelings

Giving expression to negative feelings is an important skill, as many of us become annoyed or displeased by the behavior of others. For example, often physicians and nurses speak to one another with a patronizing tone in their voices. Let's say you have discussed this together, but the patronizing tones continue, or a head nurse or administrator, after indicating she wants a task performed, then is upset when you perform it, or one of your co-workers doesn't finish her work assignment even though this has been discussed repeatedly, or you have had to pick up soiled dressings that were thrown on the floor after repeatedly asking the physician to put them in the paper bag. In response you could say directly to these persons, "You still have a patronizing tone to your voice when speaking to me; I feel put down and annoyed. Please try to correct this"; or "When you ask me to complete a task and I do, then you change your mind, I feel irritated. I would like you to only assign me what it is you want done"; or "When you don't complete a work assignment, especially after it's been repeated, I feel irritated with you"; or "When you throw soiled dressings on the floor instead of in the paper bag, I feel angry and put out. Please put them in the bag." Expressing negative feelings in this way pinpoints exactly what is distressing you and allows the other person to know what it is. In addition, this gives the other person a chance to respond directly to you, as there might be a reason from his or her viewpoint for the behavior. This allows for clarity of communication between two people.

"Feeling Talk"

"Feeling talk" is recognizing your feelings and sharing them with yourself and others. The more comfortable one is communicating in this manner the more places this skill can be used. At times in certain situations one's assertive choice may be not to use feeling talk. When you do choose this type of assertion, examples may include "I'm irritated with you, Dr. Taylor, as both the patient and I have waited over an hour for you past our original appointment time"; or "I'm filled with joy over your natural childbirth experience and the fact that you allowed me to share it"; or "I'm tired today"; "I'm nervous about assisting Dr. Taylor remove the dressings from her face"; "I love to work with you—we seem to complement each other well"; or "I'm annoyed that you speak to me in a patronizing way." Talking about one's own feeling, whether positive or negative, in relation to others is assertive and growth-producing for oneself and adds emotional honesty to relationships.

Protective Skills

You have to use protective skills when you have tried assertive skills and nothing has worked. Some people do not want to change their behavior regardless of the fact that it is aggressive or nonassertive. An example of this may be in the operating rooms. There are some doctors who yell and scream when things don't go right, or throw instruments. One nurse, after six months, had her fill and repeated these statements over and over, escalating her tone of voice, "I don't want to be screamed at any more (repeated). I feel put down when you continue to yell at me (repeated)." After hearing this for about three minutes, the doctor stopped screaming at her and said, "I didn't know it affected you that way. I was so upset with myself." Real-life situations don't always turn out this well; however, many do. The point is that without risking, one never knows what will be the outcome.

Precise Words

The use of precise, concise words to communicate thoughts, feelings, beliefs, and opinions facilitates assertion between nurses. This is influenced by the thoughts people have, how they become sorted out in their minds, and the words chosen to communicate. It also requires practice in consciously choosing words. This develops self-discipline and responsible self-action, as does learning to be assertive.

NONVERBAL SKILLS: ASSERTIVE BODY LANGUAGE

Often nurses become so involved in work that they forget to look directly at the person to whom they are speaking, to maintain a firm, even voice, or to stand up straight. This nonassertive body language does not enhance communications with others, even when assertive content is utilized.

In fact, numerous research studies (Wolpe, 1969; Lazarus, 1968; Serber, 1972; Hersen, 1973) on nonverbal components of assertive behavior indicate that nonverbal behavior accounts for about 65 percent of the communications occurring between people. Nonverbal behavior reflects an attitude of how one views oneself. People who observe others closely often do not listen to the message content, but react only to the nonverbal behavior that is present. For example, a nurse who lowers her head and never looks up is communicating timidity, insecurity, and anxiety. A nurse who stands erect with her shoulders back, and head raised, and makes eye contact communicates self-confidence and assurance. Patients, as well as other staff, very readily pick up nonassertive nonverbal behavior in nurses and other professionals. When insecurity and meekness are communicated by nurses, patients sick and dependent on health care professionals become anxious and restless and often reticent to participate in their own health care.

In the following interaction, a nurse is requesting a behavior change from a patient. Note the nonverbal nonassertive behaviors of the student nurse as she approaches the patient.

Nurse: *(She walks into the patient's room and stoops to drain his urine bag.)* "Mr. J., the aide has told me that you repeatedly refuse to get out of bed and walk when he asks you to." *(She glances up from her task momentarily.)*

Mr. J.: "I don't see much sense in getting out of bed. I just had an operation and I need rest."

Nurse *(Standing up to straighten covers)*: "But Mr. J., the reason we get you out of bed is so that you don't become weak from lying flat for so long. We want you to get well so you can return home." *(She looks at the bed while she says this and then looks around the room and glances back at him.)*

Mr. J.: "I'll get out of bed soon; I'm just not ready yet."

Nurse *(Leans close and glares at him)*: "The longer you lay in bed, the longer it will take you to recuperate. I don't know why we try so hard . . . if you don't get out of this bed this afternoon I'll have to tell the doctor." *(She turns, leaves, and notices she is frustrated.)*

The result: not only did the nurse become frustrated, but neither nurse or patient furthered patient recovery. In this particular instance, the student nurse went to a colleague in her assertion training course. They talked over the situation and role played with each other. The nonassertive nonverbal behaviors became obvious. Later in the morning, the student nurse tried using assertive body language, as in the following example:

Nurse *(Walking into the room and straight to the patient's bedside)*: "Mr. J., you haven't been ambulating as you were told to do. This upsets me very much. You need to get out of bed in order to get well."

Mr. J.: "But I've just had an operation! I don't feel well enough yet."

Nurse (*Leaning toward him, looking directly into his eyes, and with a pleasant, firm tone of voice*): "Mr. J., I understand that you are still feeling weak; however, the walking will help you to feel stronger and keep your muscles toned. It will help you to get out of bed."

Mr. J.: "Oh, all right. I guess I don't really feel so bad."

When the nurse used direct eye contact, an erect posture, gestures congruent with serious facial expression, and a firm but serious tone, the patient was responsive.

It is helpful for nurses to keep the following in mind when practicing or observing their own assertive nonverbal behaviors.

Physical Distance

In every culture there is a defined physical distance that is acceptable and that one is expected to maintain. Reducing or increasing this distance may make the other person uncomfortable. You may experience this for yourself by standing opposite another student and walking toward her while speaking. Notice when she moves from you or looks away, or uses other nonverbal body behavior that says you have intruded on her personal space. This is very important in the hospital environment. A nurse who stands facing the patient by the bed is acceptable, while a nurse who sits on the bed while explaining a procedure may not be seen as professional. On the other hand, a nurse who stands close to the patient to whom she is giving a back rub and uses the palm of her hand seems involved in her work and reflects more self-confidence than does a nurse who stands away from her patient and uses only her fingertips and speaks in a very soft voice.

Posture

A straight, erect posture connotes pride and confidence, while stooped shoulders convey the opposite impression. Dragging or shuffling one's feet while walking demonstrates tiredness, apathy, or disinterest. Nurses who have erect body posture let patients know they are interested and eager to help care for them.

Hand Movements

The use of hand movements can either add expression to a conversation or detract from it. Assertive hand movements accentuate what the verbal message is. For example, a nurse explaining how to use a breathing machine to the patient may add to the communication with hand gestures showing how the breath circulates and moves. Gestures may convey empathy, such as putting a hand on the shoulder of a patient, expressing sadness or connoting caring, or pointing a finger to emphasize a negative statement. On the other hand, gestures such as nervously tapping the bedside stand or gestures unrelated to the message will distract the patient.

Eye Contact

Maintaining eye contact during interactions adds personal involvement to the communication, shows interest, and reduces anxiety. A nonverbal message that is conveyed by anyone using eye contact is "I'm a neat, interesting person and am interested in what you have to say." Nurses conveying this assertive attitude become aware of an increased quality in their communication with others.

One way to fully develop this skill is to practice looking into your own eyes in a mirror. Notice what color and how attractive your eyes are. Next look into the eyes of your spouse or those of a friend. If at first this is too difficult, look at the area on the forehead between the eyebrows and drop your gaze into the eyes as you become more comfortable. Then maintain eye contact with anyone you engage in conversation with until it becomes a natural part of your repertoire.

Facial Expressions

Assertion training helps nurses express emotions in their faces, thus more effectively communicating feelings to others.

Many nurses demonstrate warmth and understanding by a smile. It seems harder, however, for nurses to allow anger or disapproval to show. Instead, many give an insincere smile that conveys a double message to others. For the most part, women have been socialized to be happy and pleasant to others and discouraged from showing any angry feelings. Nurses, too, as we have seen, have been taught that anger has no place in a nurturing profession. Consequently, in work situations nurses find themselves in a paradoxical dilemma. Many choose to turn anger inward, which punishes themselves, rather than be seen as angry and therefore "not a good nurse." In fact, to say "no" to a request is often seen in nursing as being angry and not thinking of others. For example, a nurse saying to her supervisor, "No, I will not be able to work overtime this evening" (with a smile on her face) will not be taken seriously and thereby invites her supervisor to continue asking her. This causes even more frustration for the nurse to handle. Learning facial talk congruent with the verbal message and one's feelings gives nurses permission to experience all feelings as a full human being.

Voice Fluency

A voice tone that is steady and firm conveys the message that the speaker knows what she is saying. A spark to the tone helps stimulate others to listen. Monotone voices quickly become boring. People stop listening.

Content

Know your subject matter. Then you will organize it naturally so that your speech will flow and be understood easily by others.

RATIONAL-EMOTIVE THERAPY

Rational-Emotive Therapy—R.E.T., as it is commonly called —is a cognitive behavior therapy. Assertiveness includes cognitive as well as affective and behavioral components. The cognitive aspect of assertion helps you focus and become aware of your thinking in relation to your feelings and behavior following a situation or event. Being cognizant of your thoughts helps you gain more control over your emotions. Albert Ellis (1962, 1971; Ellis and Harper, 1976) states that your control of yourself and your world begins in your head—how you think about an event or an experience determines your feelings and behavior. Such a theory implies that each of us can be responsible for how we live in the here and now. Ellis further states that instead of having a direct emotional reaction to an event, such as depression or guilt, as adults we have thoughts or beliefs that are either rational or irrational. When your thoughts are irrational, the behavior results are self-defeating emotions. What makes thoughts rational as opposed to irrational depends on what your individual life goals are and how you handle frustration. If your goals or values are to accept yourself as a person with worth in life and in your profession and social life, then self-defeating thoughts and the corresponding self-defeating emotions have no place in your life. In other words, you would value self-accepting thoughts and beliefs and want to be aware of any self-statements that put you down. Some people maintain self-acceptance as a goal for themselves, but not when they fail or become frustrated in their professional or work life. To accept oneself fully in all aspects of life requires work. Often it becomes unclear as to whether you are thinking rationally or irrationally. This is why it is important to be aware of your thoughts. In the following examples, if you don't get a job promotion, or fail an examination, or are accused wrongly by someone, it is rational to think how irritated or frustrated or inconvenienced you are and irrational to think how terrible it is you didn't get the job promotion, or how awful or miserable you are because you failed the examination, or how catastrophic for you and what an awful put-down that you weren't treated on the basis of how you are.

The theory behind R.E.T. is that events or situations that you are involved in stimulate your thoughts and influence how you feel about the event that precedes your behavior. Albert Ellis (1973) calls this the ABC theory: A meaning the activating event, B the thoughts or beliefs, and C the consequences, which are feelings elicited from your beliefs about the activating event or experience. One way to get at your irrational thoughts or beliefs is to check out what you felt about an event. If you experienced rage, guilt, depression, or despair, or yelled at or refused to consider any other alternatives or withdrew, these are clues that your thinking about an experience was irrational. If your feelings were of frustration, irritation, annoyance, sorrow, or regret, you probably were experiencing fairly rational or appropriate thoughts in terms of the event. Ellis has extended his ABC theory to include D and E. These additional points constitute a framework for intervening on irrational beliefs. D stands for disputing or challenging irrational beliefs—"Why is it so devastating that I didn't get a promotion, I can ask for another one"; or "I sure failed the examination, which I regret. I learned more about what I was tested on and I'll be able to pass it next time with some study"; "I was accused unfairly and I can tolerate it, although I don't like it; and I know it won't always happen." You will be asked to challenge your irrational beliefs in Chapter 4.

After you have disputed beliefs, D, then you reach step E, which refers to the effects of disputing beliefs. The effects are (1) cognitive, which are similar to rational beliefs, (2) emotional, meaning appropriate feelings—sorrowful, not depressed; concerned, not anxious; annoyed, not angry—and (3) behavioral, meaning you took positive action based on your wants and desires. At E, then, you continue substituting rational ideas for irrational, checking out your feelings, and take action. For example, in highly tense situations you might role-play before making a request for a promotion or for an opportunity to retake an examination.

You may ask, What does this have to do with assertiveness? Irrational beliefs and thoughts affect whether we choose assertive, nonassertive, or aggressive behavior, and whether we exercise interpersonal rights. For example, Mary, a staff nurse, is greatly bothered by indirect requests that are made in an irritated tone of voice. She is speaking to a physician when the head nurse says (in an irritated tone of voice) "Nobody is around here when I need them." Although Mary hasn't finished her conversation with the doctor and she prefers to, she stops and turns to the head nurse. This behavior Mary dislikes and wants to change.

Looking at the event and applying the ABC theory may help

Mary change her behavior. The *A,* or event, was the indirect request made by the head nurse in an irritated tone of voice. When questioned how she felt after the event, Mary noticed she began to feel guilty and then angry. This is *C.* When questioned about what thoughts Mary had after hearing the tone and message of the head nurse, she identified the following thoughts:

If I weren't talking to the physician, she wouldn't be angry.
I don't want her to be angry at me. I should be available to the head nurse at all times.
I must immediately stop what I'm doing, even if it is important, and attend to the head nurse's wants.
I am responsible to the head nurse.

After thinking about her thoughts, Mary decided the first four were irrational and the last one rational. She then began to think of ways to *D* dispute or challenge her irrational beliefs in this situation. She came up with the following challenging thoughts:

I don't make others angry—they choose that behavior themselves, so I can't take responsibility for the head nurse's angry voice tone. If she does get angry at me, I will survive.
I can't be available to the head nurse at all times, as I'm accountable for patient care, and that is what I'm discussing with the physician.
The head nurse could ask someone else to help her or wait until I am finished talking.
I need not stop immediately what I'm doing to attend to the head nurse's wants. I can control my frustrations and proceed with my decisions. I am discussing a patient with the physician and that is important.
"I am responsible to the head nurse" is a rational thought and next time I will ask what it is she wants when I finish talking.

At this point Mary might check out her feelings. If she still feels guilty, she repeats the above challenging thoughts until she no longer feels guilty.

Then she is ready for *E* and begins to substitute other rational ideas for irrational ones, like asking the head nurse to ask her directly when she wants something done. Also, she might decide to explain that when she was talking to the physician it was about patient care and she would like not to be interrupted unless it is an emergency.

Does this example help you apply Ellis's theory to any of your experiences? If not why not?

Researchers, such as Wolfe (1975) and Linehan and Goldfried (1975), and assertive trainers, such as Lange and Jakubowski (1976) and Galassi and Galassi (1977), have found support for the concept that the more participants think rationally, the more likely they will practice assertive behavior. In addition, by actively monitoring your thoughts, you will gain more self-respect and integration of assertive behavior.

You are encouraged to read the references listed to gain an understanding from different viewpoints regarding the application of rational-emotive therapy. Ellis (1960) has identified ten irrational beliefs that interfere at one time or another with a person's functioning productively. Briefly, these are:

1. It is a dire necessity to be loved and approved of by all significant others.
2. I should be thoroughly competent, adequate and achieving in all possible respects.
3. Some people are bad, wicked, or vile and should (or must) be punished.
4. If things do not go (or stay) the way I very much want them to, it would be awful, catastrophic, or terrible!
5. Unhappiness is externally caused and I cannot control it (unless I control the other person).
6. One should remain upset or worried if faced with a dangerous or fearsome reality.
7. It is easier to avoid responsibility and difficulties than to face them.
8. I have a right to be dependent and people (or someone) should be strong enough for me to rely on (or take care of me).
9. My early childhood experiences must continue to control me and determine my emotions and behavior!

10. I should become upset over my and other peoples problems or behavior.

The first three beliefs are the irrational assumptions regarding rejection, competence, and equality that affect most people (Ellis, 1975). The beliefs are expanded upon in Ellis's writings and, in terms of assertion, in Lange and Jakubowski (1976), Galassi and Galassi (1977), and in Wolfe and Fodor's article (1975).

You will note several references in this book to this chapter and also that irrational ideas are mentioned in many examples. Because irrational beliefs and ideas interfere with exercising interpersonal rights, you may need to refer to this section often for a more thorough understanding.

REFERENCES

Ellis, A. *Growth Through Reason*. Palo Alto, Calif.: Science and Behavior Books, 1971.

———. *How to Live with a Neurotic*. New York: Crown Publishers, 1975.

———. *Humanistic Psychotherapy: The Rational-Emotive Approach*. New York: Julian Press, 1973; McGraw-Hill Paperbacks, 1974.

———. *Reason and Emotion in Psychotherapy*. New York: Lyle Stuart, 1962.

Ellis, A., and Harper, R. *A New Guide to Rational Living*. North Hollywood, Calif.: Wilshire Book Co., 1976.

Galassi, M., and Galassi, J. *Assert Yourself! How To Be Your Own Person*. New York: Human Sciences Press, 1977.

Hersen, M., *et al.* "Effects of Practice, Instruction, and Modeling on Components of Assertive Behavior," *Behavior Research and Therapy*, (1973) 443–451.

Lange, A.J., and Jakubowski, P. *Responsible Assertive Behavior: Cognitive/Behavioral Procedures for Trainers.* Champaign, Ill.: Research Press, 1976.

Lazarus, A.A. "Variations in Densensitization Therapy," *Psychotherapy: Theory, Research, Practice,* 5 (1968): 50–52.

Linehan, M., and Goldfried, M. "Assertion Training for Women: A Comparison of Behavioral Rehearsal and Cognitive Restructuring Therapy." Paper presented at the Association for the Advancement of Behavior Therapy, San Francisco, 1975.

Otto, H. "The Human Potentialities of Nurses and Patients," *Nursing Outlook,* 8 (1965) 32–35.

Serber, M. "Teaching the Nonverbal Components to Assertive Training," *Journal of Behavior Therapy and Experimental Psychiatry,* 2 (1972): 253–254.

Wolfe, J.L. "Short-term Effects of Modeling/Behavior Rehearsal—plus—Rational Therapy, Placebo, and No Treatment on Assertive Behavior." Doctoral Dissertation, New York University, 1975.

Wolfe, J.L., and Fodor, I. "A Cognitive-Behavioral Approach to Modifying Assertive Behavior in Women," *The Counseling Psychologist,* 5 (1975): 45–52.

Wolpe, J. *The Practice of Behavior Therapy.* New York: Pergamon Press, 1969.

4 Becoming Assertive: How To Do It

This chapter is designed to incorporate the learning of assertive skills for the student by a self-help model. Reading the preceding chapters is necessary background to the following self-help model. An outline of the steps may help you in referring to specific assertive behavior.

SELF-HELP: ASSERTIVE MODEL

Step I   Learn Background for Assertive Behavior
          Exercise: Read Chapters 2,3,7
          Application: Study Them
Step II   Differentiate Assertive, Nonassertive, and
              Aggressive Behavior
          Exercise: Read Definitions
          Application: Answer Questions
          Exercise: Read Contrasts
          Application: Answer Questions
Step III   Identify Interpersonal Rights
          Exercise: Make a List of Your Rights
          Application: Answer Questions
Step IV   Review Assertive Behavior Ideas
          Exercise: Read "Assertive Behavior: Ideas to
              Keep in Mind"
          Application: Answer Questions

Level Risks at Work
Application: Answer Questions
Exercise: Identify a Specific Assertion Area
at Work
Application: Answer Questions

Now complete the following steps to becoming assertive. It is suggested that you spend a couple of hours twice a week or for five weeks block off two days. Do the exercises in order as described and answer the questions. Do not read ahead. If you need more time do not hesitate to take it; however, it is reading and practicing that help change behavior, not thinking about changing behavior. If friends have learned assertion or are reading this same book, it is helpful to spend time role playing specific situations together.

Step I Learn the Background for Assertive Behavior

Exercise: Read Chapters 2, 3, and 7.

Step II Differentiate Assertive, Nonassertive, and Aggressive Behavior

Exercise: Read out loud the following definitions:

Assertive behavior is

That type of interpersonal behavior in which a person stands up for her or his own legitimate rights in such a way that the rights of another are not violated. Assertive behavior is a direct, honest, and appropriate expression of one's feelings, opinions, and beliefs. High-quality assertion also includes an empathic component that shows some consideration, but not deference, for the other person.

Nonassertive behavior is

That type of interpersonal behavior which enables the person's rights to be violated in one of two ways:
(a) The person violates her or his own rights when she or

he permits herself or himself to ignore personal rights that
are actually very important to her or him, or,
(b) the person permits others to infringe on her or his
rights. Nonassertive behavior pays off by enabling the
individual to avoid potentially unpleasant conflicts with
others; however, various unpleasant internal consequences such as hurt feelings and lowered self-esteem are
likely to occur.

Aggressive behavior is

That type of interpersonal behavior in which a person
stands up for her or his personal rights in such a way that
the rights of another person are violated. The purpose of
aggressive behavior is to dominate, humiliate, or put the
other person down rather than to simply express one's
honest emotions or thoughts (Jakubowski-Spector, 1973).

Application: Answer Questions
1.   Do you agree with these definitions? If not, why not?
2.   Think of examples to go with these definitions. Do you
remember walking away from a situation when you could not
think how to respond without exploding in anger? Or thinking
of a response two to six hours later or even the next day?

Exercise: Read the following situation and analyze players as to
assertive, aggressive, or nonassertive behavior.

Jane was swimming laps in a community pool when she
heard an infant cry. When the cry became louder Jane
stopped and observed the following: A woman swim instructor was teaching mothers and preschool children to
swim. One mother was sitting at the side of the pool,
dressed, and facing her was the swim instructor with her
(the woman's) infant in both hands. The swim instructor
plunged the infant under the water three times and said to
the mother, "See how much he likes it." When brought up
from under the water, the baby coughed and then cried.

The pitch of the cry was loud and the tone one of powerlessness. The infant was then submerged again, brought up coughing and crying in a helplessness tone.

Jane, swimming nearby, became upset, then angry, and decided to say something. Jane swam over near the swim instructor and said, "The baby seems afraid of the water. Perhaps there is a way to teach him to swim without scaring him." The swim instructor looked at her and said, "Who are you? I am the swim instructor." Then she moved away with the infant and attached the baby's hands around a hula hoop that was in the pool. She then turned the hula hoop around in a circle and again the baby's head was under water. When she brought him up he again was loudly protesting by crying. All this time the mother sat at the side of the pool and watched.

Application: Answer Questions
1. Who in this example was assertive?
2. Who in this example was aggressive? With whom?
3. Who exhibited nonassertive behavior?
4. What basic rights were involved? (See pp. 26-27.)

Exercise: Read the contrasts out loud (Alberti and Emmons, 1974, pp. 4-8)

CONTRASTS*
Non-Assertive, Aggressive, Assertive

Non-Assertive Behavior (As Actor)	Aggressive Behavior (As Actor)	Assertive Behavior (As Actor)
Self-denying	Self-enhancing at expense of another	Self-enhancing
Inhibited, hurt, anxious	Expressive- Depreciates others	Expressive- Feels good about self

*From *Your Perfect Right: A Guide to Assertive Behavior* (second edition), By Robert E. Alberti and Michael L. Emmons. Copyright © 1974. Reprinted by permission of the publisher, Impact Publishers, Inc., San Luis Obispo, California, 93406.

Allows others to choose for him	Chooses for others	Chooses for self
Does not achieve desired goal	Achieves desired goal by hurting others	May achieve desired goal
Guilty or angry	Self-denying	Self-enhancing
Depreciates actor	Hurt, defensive, humiliated	Expressive
Achieves desired goal at actor's expense	Does not achieve desired goal	May achieve desired goal

Application: Answer Questions
1. Which behavior do you recognize in yourself? In others?
2. Which behavior style do you choose most often? In which areas: for example, work, social life, with friends or strangers?

Step III Identify Interpersonal Rights

Exercise: Make a list of your basic human rights—begin your list with "I have a right to."

Application: Answer Questions.
1. Did you identify mostly personal or professional rights?
2. Was it comfortable to use "I" when identifying your rights?
3. What rights do others have?
4. Do you ever find yourself denying your rights? If so what are you thinking or saying to yourself? (Refer to Chapter 12.)

Exercise: Read the following situation:
A patient who was nine months pregnant was admitted in active labor. After one of her labor pains, she said to the nurse:

Patient: I am so glad I took the natural childbirth classes. The breathing is helping me control the pain and I am certainly not afraid and look forward to seeing my baby born naturally.

Nurse: That's great. I'm happy for you.

Several labor pains and ten minutes later a doctor enters and says to the nurse:

Doctor: Prepare Mrs. S. for a caudal. (Spinal anesthetic)

Nurse: All right. (She gets tray, prepares the patient, and doctor gives the caudal.)

Patient never questions treatment nor does the nurse nor does anyone explain to the patient what is happening.

After the procedure, the patient says to both, "Will this procedure interfere with me having natural childbirth? Earlier I told the nurse how excited I was to be able to give birth naturally."

Application: Answer Questions
1. Who was assertive?
2. Who was nonassertive? Or aggressive?
3. What interpersonal rights were involved for the patient, nurse, and physician?

Step IV Review Assertive Concepts

Exercise: Read out loud "Assertive Behavior: Ideas to Keep in Mind" (Manderino, 1974). When reading sit erect, use a firm voice tone and any relevant facial or hand gestures to emphasize the content of ideas.

ASSERTIVE BEHAVIOR: IDEAS TO KEEP IN MIND
1. Assertive behavior is often confused with aggressive behavior; however, assertion does not involve hurting the other person physically or emotionally.
2. Assertive behavior aims at equalizing the balance of power, not in "winning the battle" by putting down the other person or rendering him or her helpless.
3. Assertive behavior involves expressing my legitimate rights as an individual. I have a *right* to express my own wants, needs, feelings, and ideas.
4. Remember: other individuals have a right to respond to my assertiveness with their *own* wants, needs, feelings, and ideas.
5. An assertive encounter with another individual may involve negotiating an agreeable compromise.
6. By behaving assertively, I open the way for honest relationships with others.

7. Assertive behavior not only is concerned with *what* I say but *how* I say it.
8. Assertive words accompanied by appropriate assertive "body language" make my message clearer and more effective.
9. Assertive body language includes the following:
   a. Maintaining direct eye contact.
   b. Maintaining an erect posture.
   c. Speaking clearly, audibly, and maintaining a firm voice tone.
   d. Making sure you do not have a whiny quality to your voice.
   e. Using facial expressions and gestures to add emphasis to your words.
10. Assertive behavior is a skill that can be learned and maintained by frequent practice.

Discussion Questions:
1. Do you agree with these ideas? Disagree?
2. Do you have any others to add?

Step V: Cope with Anxiety

Exercise: Now measure your individual level of calmness or tension by using the "Subjective Units of Discomfort Scale" (Wolpe, 1969). This scale, commonly called SUDS, ranges from 0 to 100 points representing various states of calmness to extreme tension. To rate your level of SUDS close your eyes and imagine how and where you would feel perfectly relaxed—on the beach, taking a warm bath, in the mountains, listening to music, or before falling asleep. This state for you is rated "0" SUDS. Now imagine a situation where your anxiety is highest—presenting a paper to a large group of nurses at the American Nurses Association, being the only nurse in the emergency room handling two serious accidents, having a physician criticize you in front of a patient, or observing an automobile accident involving a friend. Rate this state at "100" SUDS.

Stop here and determine on a scale of 0-10-20-50-70-100 where your SUDS measure is at present. Notice also any physiological factors that indicate anxiety, such as fast breathing, heart rate, headache, or sweaty hands. Of course, your ratings are purely subjective and a 30 on another person's scale would mean something different than the 30 on your scale. However, your scale will help you become more aware of your body state at a given moment. Be sure to choose only one number to indicate your anxiety level, that is, 30 rather than between 20 and 40. The more often you choose SUDS numbers the easier it will become to discriminate and be aware of body calmness and tension.

Application: Answer Questions
    1. What did you learn about yourself?
    2. Which physiological factors did you experience?

Exercise: Make SUDS Diary for the week when you apply assertive skills. Fill in the diary below each time you practice assertive behavior.

SUDS Diary
NAME _____

Time	SUDS	Situation	Describe Anxiety

Remember, only you know your feelings and how relaxed or anxious you are in a situation. It takes time to identify and reduce anxiety so compliment yourself often to reinforce your decision to keep the diary.

Application: Answer Questions
   1.   What did you learn new about your self and anxiety?
   2.   What specific areas do you have more anxiety about?

Exercise: Learn to Relax

Often nurses and other persons are not aware of anxiety until their level is extremely high. At this point their ability to handle the situation or diminish their anxiety is nil. Since high levels of anxiety reduce reasoning powers and incoming information is often distorted, it is helpful to maintain low levels of tension and practice relaxation to prevent higher levels of anxiety from occurring. When you are highly anxious, you are inhibited from saying what you want to say. Relaxation, like assertive behavior, is a skill that must be practiced to be learned. Learning to systematically relax muscles helps you cope with stress and reduces anxiety. Jacobson (1938) states that you cannot be tense and relaxed at the same time and recommends regular practice, twenty minutes a day, to learn deep muscle relaxation.

Relaxation skills help in asserting oneself in stressful situations as one can stop, relax, and take slow breaths before confronting an angry supervisor or a screaming physician.

Tape record, or choose a person to read the following instructions (Jacobson, 1938):

Close your eyes, lie on the floor, or get comfortable in a chair and relax. Allow yourself to breathe deeply.
Concentrate on the muscle groups as presented, one at a time.
Tense the muscles as listed below for 3 to 7 seconds and then let relax completely for 20 to 30 seconds before proceeding to the next group of muscles.

Specific Instructions:
Tense the muscles in your forehead—move your eyebrows to your hair line, relax.
Tense the muscles in your eyes by closing your eyes tightly, relax.
Tense the muscles in your nose by wrinkling it.
Tense the muscles in your lips and lower face by pressing your lips together tightly and forcing your tongue against the top of your mouth.

Tense the muscles in your jaw by clenching your teeth together.

Tense the muscles in your neck by attempting to look directly above you.

Tense the muscles in your shoulders and upper back by shrugging your shoulders.

Tense the muscles in your right hand by making a fist.

Tense the muscles in your right upper arm. Bend your arm at the elbow and make a muscle.

Tense the muscles in your left hand by making a fist.

Tense the muscles in your left upper arm. Bend your arm at the elbow and make a muscle.

Tense the muscles in your chest by taking a deep breath and holding it.

Tense the muscles in the small of your back by arching up your back.

Tense the muscles in your abdomen by either pushing those muscles out or pulling them in.

Tense the muscles in your buttocks and thighs by pressing your heels into the floor.

Tense the muscles in your ankles and calves by pointing them away from your body.

Now breath deeply, taking in air by pushing out your abdomen and exhaling slowly. Twelve times.

Now imagine yourself in a pleasant scene, such as lying in the sun at the beach or bathing or being massaged—this is your natural assertive body state.

Now you are relaxed and in a moment I will ask you to open your eyes. When you do you will be alert, yet relaxed. I will count backwards from five to one. When I reach one, you will open your eyes: 5 . . . 4 . . . 3 . . . 2 . . . 1—and slowly sit up.

As you practice this daily, record a SUDS rate before you begin. Practice one week with the tape in which muscles are tensed and relaxed once, then one week just relaxing muscles, and then try to relax individual muscles that are not being used—deep breathes before giving a talk, shoulder muscles while driving a car, leg and foot muscles while sitting in a chair. Compare SUDS before and after.

Application: Answer Questions

1. Were you at ease during this exercise? If not, explain what was uncomfortable for you: thoughts, feelings, breathing.

2. Did you have more difficulty relaxing certain muscles than others? Which ones were they?

Step VI Build a Positive Belief System

Exercise: I Need . . . .

Write down three or more items or things you need. For example:

I need . . . (vacation)
I need . . . (more money)
I need . . . (more help on my floor)

Now read them to yourself outloud and think about them for two minutes. Now cross off "need" and write in the word "want."

Again read these three things to yourself and think about them.

I want . . . (vacation)
I want . . . (more money)
I want . . . (more help on my floor)

Application: Answer Questions

1. Any changes in your attitude when the word "need" was changed to "want"?

2. Any changes in obtaining the item when the word "need" was changed to "want"?

3. What interpersonal rights are reinforced, if any?

Exercise: Write down three or more things you have to do. For example:

I have to . . . (go to work)
I have to . . . (work every weekend)
I have to . . . (always work for others)

Now read these "I have to's" out loud and think about them for two minutes. Now cross off the word "have" and replace it with "choose" so your list reads

I choose to . . . (go to work)
I choose to . . . (work every weekend)
I choose to . . . (work for others)

Application: Answer Questions
  1. When you crossed out "have" and wrote "choose" did you notice any difference in your feelings?
  2. Did you choose to do what you listed? If not what other choices can you make?

Exercise: Make a list of at least five thoughts or beliefs you hold as

1. A staff nurse of administrators, head nurses, or supervisors
2. A nurse administrator, head nurse, or supervisor of staff nurses
3. A nurse of physicians
4. A nurse as you believe physicians perceive you

Application: Answer Questions
  1. Look at your beliefs or thoughts on each list. Are more of them rational as opposed to irrational? (Refer to Chapter 3.)
  2. Keeping in mind that irrational self-messages cause you to feel anxious, depressed, or hopeless, which of these beliefs or thoughts benefit you as a person? As a member of a professional group? Which ones impede you?

Exercise: Choose three irrational beliefs from the above list. Write them again. Now write down challenges to these irrational beliefs by asking yourself the following questions about each irrational belief and write the answer.

1. Is this always true or only at present?
2. What is the evidence?
3. If it is true what's the worst that can happen?
4. Can I handle it? How does it affect me?
5. Am I worthless or no good because of this thought?

For example:

Irrational—Staff nurses occupy inconsequential positions.

Challenges (answers to above questions):

1. This seems true now but not always.
2. This particular staff nurse I'm thinking about didn't keep the lights answered on the floor.
3. Patients then had to wait before they could be cared for; some patients got visitors to help them; others had to help themselves; some cried.
4. Yes, I can handle it but I want things to go well on that floor as I'm in charge. It affects me when patients complain to me about the floor. Things should go well; when they don't this takes my time.
5. I don't like to think these thoughts as I then feel annoyed that I have to be doubly responsible for patient care. I don't want to feel that way as I get more angry and then don't feel good about myself. This is ridiculous as I have worth. It was the staff nurse who didn't answer the lights. Why do I think staff nurses are perfect or for that matter why do I think I need to direct a perfectly run hospital floor.

Rational—When I feel angry because things aren't going perfectly it seems to me staff nurses are inconsequential. In reality staff nurses care for patients on an eight-hour basis and much of patient care is based on their observation and expertise of reporting. My ability to be a charge nurse rests on how they take care of patients. Staff nurses hold a responsible job and are competent. They are not perfect.

Application: Answer Questions

1. Were the three irrational beliefs you chose similar in any way? What way? Repeat the challenges until you are convinced.

2. Did you convince yourself with your logical challenges or did they merely sound more acceptable to you? If not convinced, why not?

3. After disputing and changing the belief or thought from irrational to rational what did you feel?

Exercises: Write a situation that happened at work which you would like to have handled in an assertive fashion rather than with resulting feelings of depression or anger.

Now list the thoughts you had at the time of this situation and as you rethink it.

Look to see if you listed any feelings. If so cross them off the list.

Decide which thoughts are rational (what you wanted or desired) and which thoughts were irrational (more demands or commands that elicit angry, depressed, hopeless feelings).

Now challenge your irrational thoughts by asking yourself the following questions:

1. Is this always true or only at present?
2. What is the evidence?
3. If it is true what's the worst that can happen?
4. Can I handle it? How does it affect me?
5. Am I worthless or no good because of this thought?

Write down your challenges to each of your irrational thoughts. (Refer to Chapter 3 or Chapter 7 for additional help).

Application: Answer Questions

1. After you challenged your irrational beliefs, how did you feel?

2. Could you imagine repeating the same situation and handling it in an assertive manner?

3. Can you now label parts of the situation in terms of Ellis's ABC therory? What is the A, or event? What were the beliefs? And what were the resulting consequences to your feelings and behavior?

Step VII Refusing Requests

Exercise: Stand and look into your eyes in a mirror and practice saying "no." Use different voice tones and vary your body posture from slumping to standing erect. Feel angry or irritated and say "no." Now feel at peace and say "no."

Application: Answer Questions

1.   Were you comfortable maintaining eye contact with yourself? If not, why not?
2.   When you got angry did you maintain eye contact with yourself?
3.   How did you feel raising your voice and saying "no"?
4.   Did you smile when you said "no"?

Exercise: Read out loud "Refusing Requests: Ideas to Keep in Mind" (Manderino, 1974; modified by Herman, 1977). When reading maintain an erect posture and use a clear, firm voice tone.

REFUSING REQUESTS: IDEAS TO KEEP IN MIND

1.   I have a *right* to say no.
2.   I deny my own importance when I say yes and I really mean no.
3.   Saying no does not imply that I reject another person whether a patient, nurse, or physician—I am simply refusing a request.
4.   When saying no, it is important to be direct, concise, and use an "I" message.
5.   If I really mean to say no, I am not swayed by pleading, begging, cajoling, compliments, or other forms of manipulation.
6.   I may offer reasons for my refusal, but do not get carried away with numerous "excuses."
7.   I do not become overly apologetic; this can be offensive.
8.   I demonstrate assertive body language:
     a.   Maintain direct eye contact.
     b.   Maintain an erect body posture.
     c.   Speak clearly, audibly, and maintain a firm voice tone.
     d.   Do not whine or have an apologetic tone to my voice.
     e.   Make use of appropriate gestures and facial expression for emphasis.
9.   Saying no is a skill that can be learned.
10. Saying no and not feeling guilty about it can become a habit—a habit that can be very growth enhancing.

Application: Answer Questions
1. Do you disagree with any of the above ideas?
2. Do these ideas follow the scripts in Chapter 5?

Exercise: Take your SUDS rating. Practice behavior rehearsal by role playing the assertive model in the scripts in Appendix A and saying "no."

Turn to Appendix A and begin with the scene. Read the actors' or actresses' parts out loud, cover up the assertive model answer with a slip of paper and respond. Write your response. At the conclusion of the scene, give yourself feedback using "Refusing Requests: Ideas to Keep in Mind." Tell yourself just what you did well and then how you could improve.

Another option is to cover the assertive model's answer with a slip of paper and tape record your response. Then critique yourself using "Refusing Requests: Ideas to Keep in Mind." This method of practicing helps you hear inflections in your voice, whether you are fluent, the pitch and tone of your voice.

At this stage it is extremely helpful to obtain one or two friends who are interested in role playing. One person can be a coach and use "Refusing Requests: Ideas to Keep in Mind" from which to make positive and needs-to-improve comments. You practice enacting the role of assertive model and a friend can be the actress. Try some of the scripts in Appendix A first and then improvise scenes. You can then switch roles so that you each have a chance to be the coach (as one becomes more assertive by observing the other's verbal and nonverbal behavior) and a chance to be the actress. The actress should try nonassertive or aggressive responses to experience those roles. After each role play the coach asks the assertive model what was done well and what needed improvement and then gives her or his positive and needs-to-improve feedback using the "Ideas to Keep in Mind" list.

Application: Answer Questions
1. What was helpful in this exercise? Or not helpful?
2. What thoughts did you have as you prepared to role play?
3. What did you learn from role playing?
4. Were the structural scripts or the ones you improvised more useful?
5. What was your SUDS rating?

Step VIII Making Requests

Exercise: Make a list of "I wants." Now look in your eyes in the mirror and say out loud what "I want." Maintain eye contact and do not smile.

Application: Answer Questions
1. Did you come up with a list of "I wants"?
2. Was it hard to maintain eye contact with yourself?
3. What were your thoughts as you proceeded to ask yourself for what you wanted?

Exercise: Read out loud "Making Simple Requests: Ideas to Keep in Mind" (Manderino, 1974; modified by Herman, 1977). Maintain a firm voice tone and an erect body posture.

MAKING SIMPLE REQUESTS: IDEAS TO KEEP IN MIND

1. I can identify what I want—I want a Sunday off; I want to give a report.
2. I have a *right* to make my wants known to others.
3. I deny my own importance when I do not ask for what I want.
4. The *best* way to get exactly what I want is to ask for it directly.
5. Indirect ways of asking for what I want may not be understood; for example, complaining of a sore back rather than asking for a back rub, or complaining about having to give seven patients complete bed baths rather than asking the head nurse for additional help.
6. I demonstrate assertive body language:
   a. Maintain direct eye contact.
   b. Maintain an erect body posture.
   c. Speak clearly, audibly, and maintain a firm voice tone.
   d. Do not whine or have pleading voice quality.
   e. Make use of appropriate gestures and facial expression for emphasis.
7. Asking for what I want is a skill that I can learn.

8. Directly asking for what I want can become a habit with many pleasant rewards.

Application: Answer Questions
1. Do you disagree with any of the above ideas? Which ones?
2. How do these ideas follow the scripts in Chapter 5?

Exercise: Take your SUDS rating. Practice Behavioral Rehearsal by role playing the scripts in Appendix A or by making up your own scripts to ask for something. Refer to page 69 for further ideas on how to practice.

Application: Answer Questions
1. What was helpful in this exercise? Or not helpful?
2. What thoughts did you have before doing the behavioral rehearsal? Were they beneficial to you or a hinderance?
3. What did you learn?
4. What actors or actresses did you use if you improvised scripts?
5. Was it easier to make request of someone you knew or didn't know?
6. What was your SUDS rating? Was it higher than when you practiced refusing requests? Was it lower after practice?

Step IX Asking for a Change in Behavior

Exercise: Read out loud "Requesting a Change in Behavior: Ideas to Keep in Mind" (Manderino, 1974; modified by Herman, 1977).

REQUESTING A CHANGE IN BEHAVIOR: IDEAS TO KEEP IN MIND

1. I have a *right* to let others know that their behavior bothers me. I also have a right to ask them to modify their behavior.
2. When I do not exercise this right I deny the importance of myself as well as the relationship.
3. Follow this important four-step procedure (Bower and Bower, 1973):
    a. Describe the behavior that I see and/or hear in the other

person. It is important that I use descriptive rather than labeling words. For example, "I notice you have been leaving your dirty laundry all over the room. . . ." rather than "You are an inconsiderate slob!"

b. *Express* the feelings you experience as a result of the other person's behavior. For example, "I feel angry and resentful when you leave your dirty laundry all over the room."

c. *Ask* for a specific change in behavior. For example, "I would like you to keep your dirty laundry in the closet. Are you willing to do this?"

d. Consequences are then spelled out.
Positive consequences are given first—"When your clothes are put away I feel more like living with you" or "I want to continue living with you and this would make it easier for me." Negative consequences are given if after giving positive consequences you notice the same behavior is continuing—"If you continue to scatter your dirty laundry all over the room, I will sweep it all underneath your bed or I will put it in a plastic bag in the garage."

4. Remember to demonstrate assertive body language:
a. Maintain direct eye contact.
b. Maintain an erect body posture.
c. Speak clearly and audibly.
d. Do not whine.
e. Make use of gestures and facial expressions for emphasis.

5. Giving other people direct messages about how their behavior affects you is a skill that can be learned.

Application: Answer Questions
1. Do you disagree with any of the ideas? Which ones?
2. Did you find yourself missing any of the steps? Which ones?

Exercise: Take your SUDS rating. Practice Behavior Rehearsal by using the scripts in Appendixes or making up your own. Refer to page 69 for further ideas on how to practice.

Application: Answer Questions
  1. What was helpful about the experience? Or not helpful?
  2. Compare your SUDS rating with those of the two previous exercises. Is it higher, lower, or the same?

Step X Self-Affirming Assertions

Exercise: Make a list of your personal or professional strengths (Otto, 1965), assets, or potentialities. Try to list twenty or more.

Application: Answer Questions
  1. Was this a simple task for you?
  2. Can you think of any additional strengths?
  3. What areas were your strengths in?
  4. If you listed any problems—cross them out now.

Exercise: Read the list out loud to yourself and stop and clap or compliment yourself if you are specifically proud of one or more assets.

Application: Answer Questions
  1. Were you comfortable reading your assets and gaining approval from yourself?
  2. What thoughts were you aware of during this exercise?

Exercise: Do a SUDS rating. Now give yourself five sincere compliments and practice receiving them, that is, say "Thank you" or "I agree" or "Thanks for noticing." As the last compliment you might thank yourself for persevering through this self-help chapter. Take another SUDS rating.
  This exercise may also be done with friends. Everyone would give each other a compliment and in addition practice accepting the compliment.

Application: Answer Questions
  1. Are you more comfortable exchanging caring assertions with yourself, or another individual, or in a small group context?
  2. Was it easier for you to give the caring assertions or to receive them?

3. Did your SUDS vary with giving or receiving caring assertions?

4. Was your SUDS score lower for this exercise than the previous one?

Exercise: Think positive thoughts about yourself for three minutes. Count them. Say the thoughts out loud. Again think positive thoughts for three minutes. Count them again.

Application: Answer Questions

1. How did you feel when you focused only on positive thoughts for three minutes?

2. How do you feel about yourself now?

3. Did you have more positive thoughts the second time you practiced?

Step XI   Develop Group- and Self-Reinforcement Support Systems

Exercise: Read and fill out the following form with names of people in your life who provide you with the specific support in your relationship with them. Think of family, friends, neighbors, work associates, or acquaintances. Focus on individuals who provide you with a single special resource.

Supportive Functions	*People*
1. *Intimacy:* People who provide you with closeness, warmth, and acceptance. You can express your feeling freely and without self-consciousness. People whom you trust and who are readily accessible to you.	_____ _____ _____ _____ Total _____ _____ _____
2. *Sharing:* People who share your concerns because "they are in the same boat," or in similar situations. People who are striving for similar objectives, such as colleagues, co-workers. People with whom you share experiences, information, and ideas. People with whom you exchange favors.	_____ _____ _____ _____ Total _____ _____ _____ _____

3. *Self-Worth:* People who respect your competence in your role as manager. People who understand the difficulty or value of your work or performance in that role. People whom you respect that can recognize your skills.

_____
_____
_____ Total _____
_____
_____
_____

4. *Assistance:* People who provide tangible services or make resources available. People who don't just lend a hand but whose assistance is not limited by time or extent of help. People you can depend on in a crisis.

_____
_____
_____ Total _____
_____
_____
_____

5. *Guidance:* People who provide you with advice and methods to solve problems. People who mobilize you to take steps toward solving problems, achieving goals, and otherwise taking actions.

_____
_____
_____ Total _____
_____
_____

6. *Challenge:* People who make you think. People who make you explain. People who question your reasoning. People who challenge you to grow.

_____
_____
_____
_____ Total _____
_____

Application: Answer Questions

1. Do you have names of people in each category? Are some categories blank? If so, why not look for people to support you in this way?

2. What other kinds of people do you need to meet to fill other functions in your human relationships?

3. Do different people provide you with different things or is one person fulfilling many resources for you?

4. Are some of these people professional friends? Mostly social?

Exercise: Make a hierarchy of situations in which to assess yourself. Begin with low- and build to high-level risks. For example, low risks might be initiating a conversation with a patient and a high risk might be asking for a raise in pay.

Application: Answer Questions
 1. Were these risks emotional or fears of losing approval or a job? Where did you learn these?
 2. How did you decide how to handle the high-level risk areas? Any alternatives?

Exercise: Write down a specific assertion you want to make at work. Write any thoughts or feelings that occur to you as you think about the assertions or risks involved. Are the thoughts rational in terms of your assertion? Are the feelings rational? If not, dispute these thoughts by writing responses to them.

Application: Answer Questions
 1. What did you learn from the above exercise?
 2. Do you obtain self-reinforcement when you look at and dispute irrational thoughts?
 3. What additional positive self-statements can you make to yourself to reinforce your maintaining assertive behavior at work?
 4. Are there some situations in which you would seriously decide not to assert yourself? List them.

REFERENCES

Alberti, R.E., and Emmons, M.L. *Your Perfect Right: A Guide to Assertive Behavior,* 2nd ed. San Luis Obispo, Calif.: Impact Publishers, 1974.

Bower, S.A., and Bower, G.H. *Asserting Yourself: Practical Guide for Practical Change.* Reading, Mass.: Addison-Wesley Publishing Co., 1976.

Ellis, A., and Harper, R.A. *A New Guide to Rational Living.* Englewood Cliffs, N.J.: Prentice-Hall, 1975.

Herman, S.J. "Differential Mutual Perceptions of Doctors and Nurses and Their Effects on Task Performance." Unpublished research paper presented at the Catholic University of America, Washington, D.C., 1972.

————. "Stereotypic Beliefs of Nurses." Paper presented at The Johns Hopkins University Assertion Training Workshop, February 1977.

Jacobson, E. *Progressive Relaxation.* Chicago: University of Chicago Press, 1938.

Jakubowski-Spector, P. *An Introduction to Assertive Training for Women.* Washington, D.C.: American Personnel and Guidance Association, 1973.

Manderino, M. *Effects of a Group Assertive Training Procedure on Undergraduate Women.* Ann Arbor, Michigan: University Microfilms, 1974.

————. (Comments on Teaching Nurses Assertiveness), *Journal of Continuing Education of Nurses.* (March-April 1976): 80−81.

Menzies, I. "A Case-Study in the Functioning of Social Systems as a Defense Against Anxiety," *Human Relations* 13 (1955): 95−121.

Otto, Herbert. "The Human Potentialities of Nurses and Patients," *Nursing Outlook,* 8 (1965) 32−35.

Phelps, S., and Austin, N. *The Assertive Woman.* San Luis Obispo, Calif.: Impact Publishers, 1975.

Salter, A. *Conditional Reflex Therapy.* New York: Creative Age Press, 1949.

Wolpe, J. *The Practice of Behavior Therapy.* New York: Pergamon Press, 1969.

————. *Psychotherapy by Reciprocal Inhibition.* Stanford: Stanford University Press, 1958.

Wolpe, J., and Lazarus, A.A. *Behavior Therapy Techniques.* New York: Pergamon Press, 1966 (Now out of print).

5 Applying Assertive Behavior: How To Be the Assertive You

The application of assertive behavior to nursing practice has unlimited possibilities. Any interaction you have with patients, physicians, laboratory technicians, aides, or other nurses has the potential to be an assertive experience with positive consequences in terms of morale and self-image.

As you become more familiar with assertive behavior, you will be able to identify where to apply it in your own specialty. The examples in this chapter collected by students and colleagues show assertive behavior to be effective in maternity, medical-surgical, cardiovascular, pediatric, psychiatric, urologic, and neurology units, in community health settings and clinics, in administration and educational settings, in patient advocacy, and in teaching rights to the patient/consumer in the health care system.

It is helpful to keep in mind that when first learning assertive behavior some interaction opportunities will be overlooked. Learning assertive behavior at times is like your first day in nursing in a hospital unit. You wonder if it will all come together in a matter-of-fact, appropriate way. It will, but this takes work and practice. Spontaneity in applying assertive behavior will occur more easily as you practice (1) differentiating assertive, aggressive, and nonassertive behavior in terms of your own human rights, and (2) clearly defining nursing content and practice for yourself.

As you learn to identify daily examples of assertive versus aggressive or nonassertive behavior more readily this will increase your use of assertive skills in everyday professional situations. When refusing or making a request professionally is based on individual rights, this helps reinforce nurses to use assertive skills.

Equally important is the fact that as nurses we have a definition of nursing and can clearly identify the tasks we are expected to perform and the skills we are expected to use. Individually, to be aware of our educational background, clinical expertise, and what is in our present job description will help immensely in using assertive behavior. For instance, a head nurse has different responsibilities and functions from a staff nurse. If a head nurse is asked to give a medication to a patient and refuses to do so, realize that giving medication is not her job but that she will give the message to the medicine nurse. Staff nurses who clearly recognize that they have different job roles and are responsible for different work loads from nurse practitioners or clinical specialists become more spontaneous in their assertive responses. In addition, nurses who can identify nursing care as opposed to medical care will be able to assert themselves more clearly and quickly in day-to-day situations involving not only colleagues but physicians as well.

Reading the following examples will increase your ideas as to where and how assertive behavior can be used in nursing practice. Notice how the assertive behavior skills build upon each other. Notice also individual difference in how nurses use assertive techniques.

REFUSING REQUESTS: SAYING "NO"

Saying "no" in a matter-of-fact manner and proceeding with one's work is not easy but essential for nurses. As we have seen, both the traditional nursing socialization process and female sex role socialization reward submissive, obedient behavior. Nurses who are decisive enough to say "no" are often considered by onlookers to be not "womanly," or aggressive or selfish. Consequently, there is often resistance from nurses to say "no" in a direct, concise manner.

Since nurses have been trained to exist only for others and not to think of themselves, it is easier to say "yes" or nothing at all rather than deal with the guilt after refusing a request of a colleague, physician, or patient. Also, since many nurses believe they occupy a position of low status particularly when compared to physicians, and are powerless in the bureaucratic system, (Herman, 1977) they tend to allow others to walk on them. Nurses who cannot say "no" only perpetuate the doormat phenomenon. When nurses act as if they have no rights this becomes an open invitation for others to take advantage.

What can nurses gain by learning to say "no"? Nurses can gain self-respect and overcome feelings of powerlessness. Anxiety decreases once saying "no" to relevant issues has been learned. Feelings of self-worth and self-power replace irrational fears and the need to be a super person to all people. You are more in control if you direct and make decisions about your life rather than letting others do it.

How can one learn to say "no"? First of all, one must learn to recognize and trust one's thoughts and feelings regarding the particular request. Requests can be reasonable as well as unreasonable, depending on the time element and people involved. The mere fact that one is asked to do this or that means another person wants something regardless of whether it is reasonable.

Nurses must decide themselves to refuse or grant the request rather than looking to others. Feelings of hesitation, being trapped, or a general nervous reaction may be clues that the request is unreasonable. Oftentimes, more information is needed before a decision about whether to say "no" can be made. Nurses who were socialized to never challenge or question may have some difficulty at first learning to assert themselves by obtaining more information. Practice will overcome this limitation.

Once a decision to say "no" is reached, it helps to practice saying simply "no," or "I do not want it," or "I cannot go with you." Many nurses (Herman, 1977) and women (Phelps and Austin, 1975) have difficulty at first saying "no" in a straightforward way. It helps to practice by yourself or in a group until the "no" is said in a firm, matter-of-fact manner. "I'm sorry" or another apology added weakens the "no" and gives the other person time to make a guilt-producing statement. Nurses who assert themselves in this way may feel strange at first, but become more in control regarding decisions they may make.

Refusing a request is particularly important when nurses have overextended their own physical energy or taken on too much reponsibility, such as being head nurse with only one aide on evenings or nights with fifty or sixty patients, or working ten days without a day off. Often one's body will physically respond with a cold or by becoming easily fatigued. It is important to listen to these signs of overwork and say "no" to requests, thereby restoring your needed energy.

Time taken to evaluate a request is often well spent. Some helpful questions to ask yourself are

What will I get out of this?
Do I want this or am I doing it to please others?

If someone does not accept your assertive "no" and you have answered the above questions, it is easier to repeat your "no" in a firm manner. Cotler and Guerra (1976) state that often one must repeat "no's" in a broken record fashion when an assertive "no" is not accepted. If a firm "no" is repeated several times even if the other person tries another manipulation, the message generally gets across.

Between Nurse and Nurse

Nurse Colleague: How about covering the floor for me between 9 and 11 p.m.? John's coming over and we'll at last have a chance to talk.

Assertive Nurse: No, I must be on my own floor at those hours.

Nurse Colleague: Well—you could just glance over every now and then as my licensed practical nurse Maria is excellent and does good work.

Assertive Nurse: No, it's too much responsibility for me to watch two floors at one time. I have many sick patients needing individualized care.

Nurse Colleague: You're right—I didn't stop to think of it that way.

Supervisor: Please send your nurse to 3W immediately—they are extremely short of help and you are such a good organizer I know you can manage without her.

Assertive Nurse: No, I cannot send my nurse to 3W. I am a good organizer, but we have eight critical patients receiving oxygen and intravenous feeding who require at the minimum the care of myself and another nurse.

Supervisor: Oh, I didn't realize you had that amount of work.

Between Nurse and Doctor

A woman eight-months pregnant came into Labor and Delivery with contractions. The doctor examined her, then called to the nurse and gave her the following instructions:

Doctor: Nurse, give Mrs. C. 50 mg Demerol to help her relax.

Assertive Nurse: I'd suggest ordering something else as Demerol is not to be given to a woman with a premature fetus. It would depress the fetus' respirations and the fetus could not take that.

Doctor: You're right, nurse. Thank you for telling me. I won't give the Demerol.

In this situation, the nurse refused the doctor's request based on her knowledge. She not only had the right to say "no," but in addition she was responsible for the patient's welfare. By asserting herself through refusing his request, she probably saved the baby's life.

Doctor: Nurse, would you get me some 2 x 2's please. (Nurse is across the room)

Assertive Nurse: No, I'm very busy right now—there are some 2 x 2's to your right on the cart.

Doctor: Okay. (He gets 2 x 2's himself)

The nurse's refusal was based on her right to finish the task at hand and also based on the right that others can help themselves in many instances.

Assertive Student Nurse: Dr. K., Mrs. M. would like to see you when you have time.

Dr. K.: Okay, thanks. While you're here you can help me with this pelvic exam.

Assertive Student Nurse: No, I don't have time right now. I'm team leader tonight and there are many things I need to get done.

Dr. K.: It won't take long.

Assertive Student Nurse: No, I don't have the time to spare, but I'll assign someone to help you.

Dr. K.: All right.

Between Student Nurse and Instructor

Instructor: Laurie, can we discuss your nurse's notes now?

Assertive Student Nurse: No. I don't have time now. But I will be finished with this fractional urine specimen in about 10 minutes. Can we talk then?

Instructor: Yes.

Assertive Student Nurse: The dermatology clinic has finished patient care today.

Instructor: Would you like to go to another clinical area?

Assertive Student Nurse: No. I would like this time to work on my paper.

Instructor: Okay, if you feel that's your priority.

Assertive Student Nurse: Yes, it is.

Instructor: Good luck working on your paper and I'll see you in class tomorrow.

The interpersonal right involved here is the right to establish a priority of needs and to meet those needs accordingly.

Instructor: There's a catheterization on Ms. Black that needs to be done. I know you are competent in that procedure. Would you do it?

Assertive Student Nurse: No, I don't have enough time. My patients are not cared for as yet.

Instructor: All right, I'll get someone else.

Nurse: Miss Smith, will you administer this medication to Mr. B.?

Assertive Student Nurse: No, you prepared the medication, I cannot give it.

Nurse: Oh, please, I've got so many medications to give out.

Assertive Student Nurse: I realize you are busy, but I legally cannot give that medication to Mr. B.

Nurse: You student nurses are sure picky. (Indirect aggression-labeling)

Another similar situation:

Student Nurse: Kathy, will you please give Mr. L. his morphine shot?

Assertive Student Nurse: No, he's your patient, you give him the shot.

Student Nurse: But I've never given him an injection before and I'm nervous.

Assertive Student Nurse: I will go with you, but you give the injection.

Between Nurse and Patient

A post-op abdominal hysterectomy patient has been in the recovery room for thirty minutes. She is still slightly drowsy.

Patient: Oh, oh, Nurse, my stomach is hurting me. Please give me something. I can't stand the pain.

Assertive Nurse: I can't give you any medicine yet because the anesthetic hasn't worn off. It would be bad for you to get more drugs on top of the ones you've already had.

Patient: Oh, but my stomach hurts. You're so mean!

Assertive Nurse: I am sorry, but I can't give you any medicine yet. When you wake up more and the anesthetic wears off, then I will be able to give you something. I can help you change your body position, that may help.

In this situation, the nurse again is responsible for the patient, and based on her nursing knowledge has the right to persist and refuse the patient's request. It becomes more difficult to say "no" when a patient is in pain, but the assertive nurse is secure in her knowledge that her refusal is best for the patient and often can use nursing care to relieve discomfort.

Assertive Student Nurse: Here is your medication Mrs. X.

Patient: Thanks. Could you just put it over there on the table. I'll take it later.

Assertive Student Nurse: No, I cannot, Mrs. S., your medication has to be taken at certain times to be effective. Your doctor has prescribed those times. It is my responsibility to see that you take your medication before I can record that you have.

Patient: I hadn't realized there was a reason why I had to take my pills at a particular time. Sure, I'll take it now.

This represents the nurse's right and obligation to others to properly carry out responsibilities.

Assertively saying "no" in these hospital incidents helped the nurse avoid becoming involved in situations she would have professionally as well as personally regretted, prevented her from being manipulated, and allowed her to make the decisions to direct her professional behavior.

MAKING SIMPLE REQUESTS: SAYING WHAT YOU WANT

Often as a nurse you need assistance in getting a patient out of bed, in finishing a work assignment because of additional admissions, in trading days off because of personal or social commitments, or for numerous other reasons. Regardless, you have a right to make a direct request of another person, understanding that he or she has the right to comply or refuse. When nurses are direct in asking what they want, others do not have to interpret what they mean. Making simple requests and beginning them with "I want" or "I would like" reinforces a basic human right to make one's wants known; for example, "I want you to order a pain medication for Miss S.," or "I would like this weekend as my days off." Hinting or indirectly talking around issues is a way of getting the other person busy at interpreting. The responsibility for getting your desires met starts with your request. "Would you help me clean the diet kitchen" is a request for help. Grumbling in report that "the diet kitchen sure is a mess" is an annoying hint. Stating "I want you to clean the diet kitchen" is an assertive request.

Making simple requests sounds simple. It is. However, when the nurse, her colleagues, or the physician do not know what they want, requests are often made indirectly in the hope that the other person may suggest or decide what is wanted. This ambiguous communication gives neither party full permission to his or her rights as a person or a chance to maintain self-esteem because neither admits "I don't know what I want." Instead it creates a subtle game between the players. The results are not only seriously impeded communication between two professional people but lowered self-esteem for both.

How does this happen between doctors and nurses? Traditionally, the physician has total responsibility for making decisions regarding management of his patients' medical care. He collects data from the patient through various history-taking procedures, performs physical examinations, interprets laboratory findings, and receives consultation from other physicians.

The nurse provides care and nurturance to patients but also observes and describes the daily behavior patients present. Nurses gather the data about patients on a day-by-day basis to present to doctors for their decisions or diagnoses. Traditionally, nurses were and often still are taught to pretend that only doctors could make decisions as to the final diagnosis. However, most decisions made today by nurses are management as well as nursing decisions. More recently, nurse practitioners have made diagnoses, working closely with physicians rather than alone. Laws presently limit nurses from the independent practice of nursing skills in many states. Nurses also limit themselves in making simple requests. Actually, doctors often indirectly ask for recommendations from nurses regarding patient care. Because of this professional model and lack of practice the nurse often apologizes when attempting to request a medication for a patient or disguises the fact that she is making a request as she was educated to present only observations. The usual nurse rationale is that if physicians are indirect how can we nurses who are dependent on medicine be direct? Indirect communication is the end product. For example:

Nurse, talking to Dr. Willow, "Miss Smith, whose mother died today from a car accident, can't sleep and complains of pain." This statement is nonassertive. Instead of a direct request, the nurse relates pertinent observations and it is confusing as to what the nurse wants from the doctor:

1. a sleeping or pain medication order?
2. some consultation on how to talk to Miss Smith regarding the death of her mother?
3. encouragement for herself as the nurse is overwhelmed by the patient's tragedy?

This indirectness allows doctors to choose from the many alternatives offered by the nurse and continue the problem-solving process until a decision is reached. Leonard Stein (1968) refers to this indirect communication as the doctor-nurse game, in which both players must play the same way for either to maintain self-esteem. The cardinal, unspoken rule is that the nurse must be able to make a recommendation without appearing to, and the doctor must be able to obtain recommendations without directly asking for them. If both doctor and nurse happen to play the game at the same time and do well they still lose, since neither has communicated as a total individual person (which adds to self-worth) but both have colluded with each other. If the doctor plays and the nurse does not, they both lose, and if the nurse plays and the doctor does not, they both lose. In these examples it is difficult to tell who is taking responsibility and vagueness is the result. The nurse can neither reward herself by feeling satisfaction nor expect acknowledgment from the physician for her problem-solving ability, and vice versa.

Both nurse and physician are using nonassertive behavior in which they both avoid and deny that either firmly advocates a recommendation or direction. An assertive request, on the other hand, provides clarity as to what is wanted and who is asking for it. Using "I" messages indicates who is responsible for the request.

An assertive nurse making a simple request in the same situation might say to Dr. Willow:

> I would like an order for a sleep and pain medication for Miss Smith. I notice she is suffering from her auto injuries more this evening and in addition she has been quite upset about her mother's death. I have talked with her about this and now it is obvious she is quite exhausted both physically and emotionally.

In this assertive request the nurse was clear about what she wanted for the patient and could also present her observations and other interventions. Her trust of herself was evident in the way she stated her request. Her directness allows the physician to agree, disagree, or to talk further considering a decision. When nurses use an assertive approach, clarity with staff and physicians is maintained. On the other hand, many physicians nonverbally ridicule or criticize nurses who speak in a firm competent voice because they are insecure with suggestions received from nurses even though they depend on them to do their work. It is hoped that this will improve as nurses continue to assert their knowledge and make requests as people who have equal rights as other staff members on the health care team.

A basic principle in making a request is to ask for exactly what you want. In other words, be direct, state specifically what you want to the person at an appropriate time. This will help avoid confusion, will ensure that your request is heard, and gives the other person the opportunity to decide whether to grant or refuse the request.

Between Student Nurse and Head Nurse

Assertive Student Nurse: Are you going to assign us a particular time for a dinner break?

Head Nurse: Yes, why?

Assertive Student Nurse: I would prefer eating later, at 5:30 p.m.

Head Nurse: All right, you may eat dinner at 5:30.

This reflects the interpersonal right of self-preferences. In this example, assertiveness resulted in a pleasant reward for the assertive nurse, without infringing on the rights of others.

Between Student Nurse and Instructor

Assertive Student Nurse: I'm not feeling well this morning and don't feel well enough to stay in clinical. I will have to go home.

Instructor: What's wrong?

Assertive Student Nurse: I feel dizzy and faint.

Instructor: Did you get any sleep last night?

Assertive Student Nurse: Yes, the same amount as I usually do.

Instructor: Did you eat breakfast?

Assertive Student Nurse: Yes.

Instructor: Well, if you're not feeling well, you should not work in the nursery.

Assertive Student Nurse: Yes, that's what I thought too.

Instructor: Okay, you can leave, but go down to sick call and get help.

Assertive Student Nurse: Yes, I will.

This reflects the interpersonal right to provide for one's optimal health status. It shows assertive behavior in approaching an instructor and stating a specific need, without being apologetic or hesitant.

Between Graduate Nurse and Head Nurse

Head Nurse: Well, Grace, how is it going?

Assertive Graduate Nurse: Ruth, are you busy right now? I'd like to talk with you.

Head Nurse: No, I'm not busy. What would you like to talk about?

Assertive Graduate Nurse: Next week when you make ward assignments could you assign me to Ward X? Working now on Ward Y is very difficult for me. I haven't had the experience and I think I can give better patient care on Ward X as I somehow have greater empathy for those patients.

Head Nurse: I'm sure I can work that out. M. has had more experience on Ward Y and she can work it next week. Maybe you could spend time with her if you aren't too busy on X next week, talking to her about Ward Y.

Assertive Graduate Nurse: That sounds fine.

In this example the nurse approached the head nurse, and using assertive body language and behavior expressed her desire to work on another ward. It is important when making a request to ask directly for what is desired. Indirect ways of asking or hints may not be understood and may leave the nurse frustrated.

Between Nurse and Head Nurse

A head nurse is talking to another R.N. about team leading (a job that is supposed to be rotated between all the T.N.s—Team Nurses—on the ward).

Head Nurse: Miss R., would you be team leader for Ward 21 this week?

Assertive Nurse: No, I'd rather not. I have been team leader twice already, while some other R.N.s have not done it at all. I understood that it was to be rotated between all R.N.s. I think someone who hasn't had it should take it before I take it again.

Head Nurse: You're right. I didn't realize that you had had it twice. I will get someone else to do it.

In this situation the head nurse made a request and the staff nurse refused based on her rights as an individual not to be treated unfairly.

Assertive Head Nurse: Will you administer the medications to all the patients tonight, please?

Staff Nurse: But the team leader usually does that.

Assertive Head Nurse: I realize that, but will you please do it tonight?

Staff Nurse: Yes.

The head nurse made a request, listened to the staff nurse, but persisted in the original request.

Between Nurse and Patient

Mr. L., a twenty-six-year-old man was undergoing X-ray treatment for testicular cancer and was discovered smoking on the ward.

Assertive Nurse: Mr. L., have you been told that you are not supposed to smoke on the ward?

Mr. L.: Oh, sure, honey, but I don't feel real well right now and the night nurse lets me.

Assertive Nurse: I understand you don't feel well, Mr. L., however smoking in bed is against hospital and ward regulations. It presents a fire hazard and is disturbing to other patients. The hospital does allow you to smoke in the corridors and I would like you to restrict your smoking to the halls. Will you please do this?

Mr. L.: Yes, I suppose I could.

Between Nurse and Doctor

The following is a request made by a nurse of a doctor to facilitate patient care and expedite the patient's return to a healthy state.

Assertive Nurse: Dr. X., I would like to speak with you for a moment, if I could.

Doctor: All right, what is it?

Assertive Nurse: My students and I had a conference yesterday and we realized that Mrs. Y. is being badly neglected. Her wound has dehisced and she is two weeks post-op. She has been up in the chair three times but has not been turning, coughing, or deep breathing regularly. She has not been eating anything except apple juice and she is still getting 20 U of NPH insulin. Without adequate protein, vitamin C, and zinc in her diet, wound healing will not be able to occur as easily and infection may set in to that open wound. Following the last culture, Pseudomonas was present in the wound. The staff tends to ignore Mrs. Y. Something really must be done.

Doctor: I guess we have really been so concerned with her cancer, that we have forgotten about any other problems that may have been developing. Thank you for bringing them to my attention. What would you suggest?

Assertive Nurse: I would suggest supplemental vitamins with zinc and a high protein dietary supplement such as Ensure. Due to her daily injection of insulin and inadequate ingestion of food, she is likely to go into hypoglycemia. Her urine, however, has been free of glucose since her surgery. We are also planning to hold a clinical care conference on her and we would like you to attend.

Doctor: Is there anything else?

The above example shows a nurse making a request of a doctor. The nurse had a specific goal in mind and acted upon it. The patient was not being cared for in a way that the nurse thought was adequate. The nurse did the research and came up with data that supported her request.

Nurses who assert themselves when making requests discover often that others are willing to fulfill them and they maintain self-respect.

ASKING FOR A CHANGE IN BEHAVIOR: SAYING WHAT YOU WOULD LIKE

Once comfortable saying "no" and making requests, nurses may combine these skills to ask a colleague, physician, or patient to change their behavior. As nurses we are often faced with reoccurring situations, as perhaps with a night nurse who has been twenty minutes late for the last two weeks. Her behavior causes you to be late in giving her evening report and late leaving the unit. You ask to speak to her alone and describe her behavior and ask her to change. You might say "You've been late the last two weeks coming to work. When this happens I feel annoyed and irritated that you are not respecting my needs, which include leaving work when my shift is finished. I would like you to be on time from now on. That way I'll feel better about working with you." Reply: "Oh, I didn't realize you felt that way and I have been sleeping late in the evenings. I'll be here on time."

This does not mean the other person must comply. Regardless, a better understanding or more agreeable terms on an issue between two people can often be negotiated to improve work or social relationships. Asking for changes in behavior and practicing the asking increases chances for more egalitarian interactions in the health care system. This has positive benefits, as professionals and patients who experience more balanced communication would feel they have more self-control. In an area in which uncertainty is always the reality, more self-control would counteract the dependency and insecurity an illness inflicts on both patients and professionals as well.

Nurses who are assertive and role model assertive behavior are inadvertently teaching direct communication to patients and other health care workers. Experiencing an effective assertive role model helps reinforce internal positive beliefs that (1) satisfactory interpersonal relationships require each person to be honest and direct, and (2) people have basic human rights.

Although the above two statements are true, it is important that you do not ask indiscriminately for changes in people's behavior. To think another nurse or a physician will make drastic personality changes is unrealistic. To ask a physician never to raise his voice, for example, if he has always functioned in this way may not work. In specific instances accepting the way others present themselves may be more assertive—depending on the situation. Remember when asking for a change you are asking for what you want. The other person may or may not decide to change. And if she or he does change, there are no other obligations or guarantees that old behavior may not occur again. When people care for each other or are working effectively they often choose to change behavior more freely.

Practicing this technique helps you increase your feelings of self-worth and self-power. Getting together the four steps (as described in Chapter 4) requires work on your part but oftentimes brings additional insights about the situation. Your efforts are reinforced by pleasant self-feelings as a result of sharing more of yourself with another person.

Between Nurse Practitioner and Nurse

A nurse practitioner was walking through the clinic and heard loud slapping noises and some crying. When she looked into the treatment room, she saw an older nurse attempting postural drainage on a ten-year-old boy. Instead of cupping her hands, the nurse had her palms flat and that was causing the slapping noise the nurse heard. The patient was periodically crying out.

Nurse Practitioner: Please step outside a minute.

Nurse: When I finish this, I'll talk to you.

Nurse Practitioner: I must see you immediately.

At this point the nurse stopped and came to the hall.

Nurse Practitioner: I noticed that your palms were flat while attempting postural drainage on the young boy. The technique accepted in this institution is to cup one's hands. It is an effective method and is more comfortable for the patient. I'll be happy to demonstrate this procedure for you.

Nurse: I don't need your help—I have been doing it this way for twenty years and will continue. (Returns to patient.)

The nurse practitioner standing in the hall was undecided whether to approach the nurse again in a firmer manner or to report the incident to the supervisor. The practitioner noticed she felt irritated that she hadn't been understood. Based on this, the nurse practitioner decided to wait until the nurse finished and talk with her again. When the nurse came out of the room, the nurse practitioner said

Nurse Practitioner: I want to talk to you for a few minutes. I understand that you have been practicing postural drainage for several years and I know from previous experience that you are a very conscientious nurse. However, the procedure for postural drainage at this hospital was revised last summer.

Nurse: Revised?

Nurse Practitioner: Yes, last summer.

Nurse: I wasn't aware of that, maybe because I was off all summer. I will think about it as I get upset and feel frustrated when the boy cries out but realize that he needs the procedure to improve. That's probably why I might have sounded sharp to you. It's difficult to help a patient but at the same time cause discomfort.

Nurse Practitioner: Yes, it certainly is. I am glad we talked.

This example illustrates direct, honest communication about the issue of postural drainage. The nurse practitioner used clear concise words, persistence in getting her point across, empathy in considering the other nurse's dilemma, made a conscious decision to continue the conversation after a space of time, and trusted her feelings that she wasn't being understood, which enabled her to continue the conversation. A conversation that began with a potential to explode in anger ended with both persons maintaining self-respect and respect of the other.

Between Nurse and Patient

Background: This patient, Mr. Horn, was a G.I. bleeder with severe hepatic failure secondary to alcohol abuse. He had been in the Medical Intensive Care Unit for approximately one week, and had been getting tube feedings as his orders were "Nothing by Mouth." He had pulled out his nasogastric tube the day before this interaction took place, and was belligerent, constantly complaining of hunger, requesting solid food, and yelling obscenities at the nursing staff.

Mr. Horn: I'm starved. They haven't fed me for a week and I want some food. Get it for me, will you?

Assertive Student Nurse: Mr. Horn, as far as I know the doctor hasn't yet ordered food for you; he's giving your stomach a rest because of the bleeding you are having. I'll ask Dr. Karn.

Mr. Horn: Okay.

(Ten minutes later)

Mr. Horn: Well, where's my food?

Assertive Student Nurse: Mr. Horn, Dr. Karn will not be on the ward for another hour, and I was unable to reach him by phone. Dr. Scott said that Dr. Karn must be the one to change the order. I will speak to him as soon as he comes up here, and we'll try to do something about this for you.

Mr. Horn: Oh, yeah. Sure. All you nurses are the same. This is a lot of shit.

Assertive Student Nurse (asking for change in behavior): Mr. Horn, I realize that you are upset and hungry; I am trying to do something for you, but I must wait for Dr. Karn. When you start yelling at me, I feel more frustrated and upset. Please stop talking to me like this.

Mr. Horn: *(Pause)* I'm sorry. I don't mean to upset you. All I want is something to eat.

Assertive Student Nurse: I know and it is hard to wait when you haven't eaten for so long.

Assertive Student Nurse: *(Twenty minutes later)* Mr. Horn, I just spoke to Dr. Karn and he has ordered some solid food for you. I'll bring you some juice now to start with, so that you can begin eating and drinking gradually.

Mr. Horn: Thank you! You're the only one up here who's listened to me!

Assertive Student Nurse: Mr. Ash, I am trying to change your shirt and you keep hitting me. When you do this you hurt my arm, and I feel annoyed. Please lie still, and don't move around while I straighten out your shirt. I want to help you—not hurt you.

Mr. Ash: *(Keeps striking out, groaning, moving in bed)*

Assertive Student Nurse: *(Student nurse with her hand on his shoulder)* Mr. Ash, you are moving around and hitting me. Just what I asked you not to do. I'm irritated, if you don't stop moving now, I will have to tie your hands down!

Mr. Ash: *(Lies still in bed)* Oh.

Assertive Student Nurse: Thank you, Mr. Ash. *(Pats his arm.)*

Between Student Nurse and Doctor

Let's look at an incident at a mental health clinic and subsequent interactions with the doctor.

Incident: A student nurse was meeting with a patient for an hour three times a week according to a contract agreement. The patient's psychiatrist came in during the last twenty minutes of one of these meetings and stated that she wanted to see the patient. The student nurse told her that their (student nurse and patient) therapy hour would be finished in twenty minutes. The doctor threw up her arms in disgust, said "huh!!" and angrily stomped out of the room.

First interaction with the doctor (first thing the next morning):

Assertive Student Nurse: Dr. Brown, I'd like to talk with you about what happened yesterday. *(Didn't wait for the doctor to answer.)* Would you like to have a list of the times I meet with L. *(patient)?*

Dr. Brown: No! I'm on a schedule and I have things I must get accomplished in a certain amount of time. When I want to see my patient I will have to take precedence over you. I'm the doctor and I'm the number one person on this team. I have responsibilities I must meet. You are just a student and you will have to accept that—that's the way it is. I'm sorry *(verbal intonation did not connote a feeling of being sorry!)* if I have to interrupt you, that's just the way it will *have* to be.

At this point the meeting was terminated—student was flabbergasted by the aggressiveness of the doctor.

Second interaction (about ten minutes later, back on the ward). Again interaction was initiated by the student.

Assertive Student Nurse: I'd like to work this problem out—if you would tell me when you would like to meet with Miss Wells, I'll work my schedule times around yours.

Dr. Brown: You don't understand! I don't have set times I can meet with her. I'm very busy, and I have to see her whenever *I* have the time. I have new admissions that come in and I don't know when that will be. I can't tell you when I will meet with my patient but again . . . when I get the time I will take precedence over you! My time is precious. I have scheduled amounts of time I must meet with my patients and if I have to interrupt you *I'm sorry*—that's the way it will have to be. *(Very angry; red face, raised voice.)*

Assertive Student Nurse: I understand that you're busy, however. . . .

Dr. Brown: I am and I can't allow you to meet with Miss Wells if I have time available. I have my responsibilities to meet and that's the way it will have to be!!

Assertive Student Nurse: Well. . . . All right.

Third interaction (several days later and planned). The student asked Dr. Brown several times for some time to talk with her. The doctor finally agreed and the following conversation ensued:

Assertive Student Nurse: Dr. Brown, I feel very unsettled by our last two conversations regarding my contract with the patient. I don't think we have sufficiently solved the problem and I would like to talk about it now. At the point things are now, it is the patient who is suffering from our disagreement. She is in the middle and is being forced to decide whom she wants to meet with and talk to. I don't think this is a decision a patient need make. I hope that you and I can work this problem out between us so that it isn't the patient who receives the brunt of the conflict.

Dr. Brown: *(Much calmer this time.)* Well, you're right, it isn't the patient's position to make a decision of whom to see. However, my point is that neither one of you can make a decision; I will decide myself.

Assertive Student Nurse: Do you understand my contractual agreement with Miss Wells and my function as a therapist?

Dr. Brown: Yes, but I am busy and will have to preempt you, if that's the only time I can see the patient. You see, I'm very busy. I have to drop everything when an admission comes in. I don't have any choice. I only have so much time during the day. If I don't see my patients x-number of hours a week Dr. Chief will be down on me.

Assertive Student Nurse: I understand that you are busy but. . . .

Dr. Brown: ... and if the Chief physician wants to see the patient when I am with her, he can preempt me. The physician takes priority though. If I don't attend to my responsibilities who will? And I am the number one person responsible.

Assertive Student Nurse: I understand you have responsibilities, but I too have responsibilities ... to the patient, to the Clinic, to the nursing staff, and to the University School. I'm not a free floating agent. I've got schedules to adhere to and specified times to meet with. ...

Dr. Brown: (interrupting; very angry with what has just been said) Look, at least I took the time to listen to you. Most doctors wouldn't even listen to what you have to say. I have been out of medical school fifteen years, I've taught at the medical school, I've been the chief attending physician, and I've had a lot of experience! You are just going to have to understand that physicians are the head of the team and are ultimately responsible. If I have to interrupt you I'M SORRY!! but that's the way it will have to be (backing away) and if my schedule demands I see the patient when you want to, I'm sorry!! And if this interferes with your plans to meet with the patient, I'm sorry! The role of the nurse is secondary to the physician. Nurses are a good source of knowledge about the patients but my time takes priority over nurses'. If you don't have a person who is the head of the team, the result is chaos! I know. I've worked where everyone on the team is equal! It doesn't work!

Assertive Student Nurse: Do you understand my position, Dr. Brown? That I have duties and responsibilities I have to accomplish. ...

Dr. Brown: Yes ... but again .... (reiteration of the same ideas)

Assertive Student Nurse: Then what can you and I do to work this problem out? I think you and I can work this out between us.

Dr. Brown: I will just have to preempt you as I said before (etc., etc.).

At this point the student nurse realized that they were at a stalemate. She could either say she would not follow the doctor's orders and continue fighting or she could decide to end the discussion. She chose to do the latter.

Result: In two subsequent meetings the student had with the patient, Dr. Brown came into the room but did not interrupt or become visible to the patient. Another time when the student nurse was chatting with another patient in the dayroom, rather than interrupt, Dr. Brown stood off to the side and softly whispered, "Are you busy seeing that patient?" The student replied "No."

The doctor's behavior thus slowly but surely did change. The student felt better about herself and relieved that her therapy hour with the patient was no longer violated. There was no verbal negotiated change, but behaviorally the physician did change the interrupting behavior.

CARING ASSERTIONS: GIVING TO SELF AND OTHERS

Nursing as a caring, nurturing profession cannot ignore the expression of feelings of affection and tenderness nurses have for one another as colleagues as well as for the patients to whom they administer.

The title of this section means being caring for oneself as well as to others. This means being cognitively assertive in caring ways, such as thinking good things about ourselves, giving ourselves compliments, treating ourselves to positive thoughts and our bodies to good physical care. Eating well, exercising, and protecting your health are other ways of caring for your self. Setting limits on work or on social activities helps you maintain a balance so that you feel cared for as you want to care for others. Giving yourself time to think, to read, or for diversions such as hiking, or going to the beach or the mountains is caring for yourself. It is extremely difficult for nurses to realize what wonderful people they are and that to remain so means we must care for ourselves well. Knowing and learning about your thoughts and feelings are additional ways to say "I care for me."

Giving personal caring in forms of tenderness and affection to others is one of the most difficult assertions to put into practice daily, according to Alberti and Emmons (1975). Many adults in work situations forget to thank others or to point out, for example, what a marvelous job a colleague did in listening to a patient and responding with emotional openness to how well the patient expressed her/himself, or that it was beautiful to understand how the patient was feeling or flattering for someone to share with you their sadness about a situation.

Nurses have more practice in this than most persons as they constantly deal intimately with people in all sorts of circumstances. What wonderful opportunities to show genuine caring outside of the steoreotypes of either romantic love or traditional sex roles. When you begin to give and share positive feelings toward others you become aware of the positive things people say about you. This begins with a personal message to a patient or colleague that conveys to them, "you are an important person to me at this time." In the hospital this occurs by a warm touch on the arm, clasping someone's hands, a warm smile, listening to what the other person says, inviting the patient to call you if she or he needs help, coming immediately when a patient calls, saying to a patient, "I'd like to help you, please let me know how I can," or "I thought about you over the weekend."

Verbalizing these thoughts and feelings to others helps patients and colleagues know you appreciate them. This is important in the work area for yourself and colleagues as well as in the healing process for patients.

Between Student and Patient

Assertive Student Nurse: I liked it when you said you especially liked to have me help with your dressing change as I was careful and tender. I appreciate your noticing particularly as it requires a lot of patience and pain tolerance on your part to undergo the treatment. You have a lot of courage.

Between Student and Nurse

Assertive Student Nurse: Thanks for supervising me while I catheterized Miss Brown. I realized you were busy but I couldn't do it alone as I hadn't taken that part of my clinical yet. I also appreciated your reminding me about the catheterized urine specimen after I had left the patient's room.

Between Nurse and Doctor

Assertive Nurse: Dr. Brown, I noticed that after you explained to Miss Geats that you had not received her message, she listened intently to your explanation about her impending surgery. Your explanation seemed to be comforting to her and your tone of voice conveyed a sincerity in wanting the patient to understand.

How wonderful for both the patient and you, that you took the time to speak in that manner to her. I admire that quality you have.

Assertive Nurse: Dr. Brown, I will finish up this treatment. I would like you to speak to Miss Miller now, she is in extreme pain and the medicine has not helped. Please see if another medication could help her.

Between Doctor and Nurse

Assertive Doctor: Nurse, I appreciate your staying with Mr. Turner after I finished his treatment the other day. He seemed upset and I noticed he responded to your touch and daily directions for his treatment very well.

Between Student and Head Nurse

Assertive Student Nurse: Miss Netts, I admired the calm manner in which you spoke to Dr. B. after the harsh tone of voice and verbal put-down he used with you. You stood your ground while at the same time remaining in control of your feelings. I noticed he even began speaking more directly and sincerely.

Head Nurse: Thanks for the compliment and for your observations. It was difficult but I feel better about myself for handling the interaction in that manner.

SPEAKING FOR OTHERS: PATIENT ADVOCACY

The role of patient advocate in nursing is very familiar and traditional. Nurses have often asserted themselves to assure that the rights of the patient are not violated when the patient cannot do so for herself or himself or if the difficulty is a staff problem that affects the patient.

To be accountable in the area of advocacy it is essential to know and understand the standards of nursing as well as the patients' bill of rights that have been established for the specific state and institution. With this legal knowledge as a base, nurses can make appropriate and reasonable assertions in behalf of the patient. It is important that patient advocacy take place only when the patient cannot speak or take care of himself. Sometimes this is a thin line, but nurses who adhere to this principle create patient involvement in their health and self-care. Patients who cannot assert themselves may be unconscious, unable to get out of bed, in a great deal of pain or discomfort, too young to realize the situation or understand its consequences, lack the ability to do problem-solving, or may be extremely anxious and insecure.

The nurse acts as an advocate when she assertively explains or gives information to patients, as when she explains a consent form or procedure. It is important to give both pros and cons regarding what the patient wants to know. If the nurse is assertively explaining a procedure, it is important that she watch and help the patient practice the same procedure. In this way assertion on the part of the patient is encouraged. The nurse may be a patient advocate to physicians, other health team members, or to social agencies. When speaking for the patient it is very important to use "I" messages to differentiate to others who is responsible for what.

Examples of Patient Advocacy

A patient was under hand-washing precautions (that is, all staff were to wash their hands before entering the room, wear rubber gloves before touching the patient, and wash their hands again upon leaving the patient's room). The student nurse was the only person following these precautions. The staff and doctors would all ignore this procedure. To protect the patient, the student nurse had the following conversation with the staff nurse in charge:

Assertive Student Nurse: Excuse me Miss White, I'd like to talk to you about something. I've noticed that I seem to be the only person on this ward who follows the hand-washing precautions for Mr. Meyer. The rest of the staff and the doctors do not.

Staff Nurse: They should. (*She turns away, giving the impression she wasn't really listening.*)

Assertive Student Nurse: Yes, everyone should, but the problem is that everyone doesn't. I think that this is annoying and I want either everyone to follow the precautions or have the basin of betadyne removed from outside his door because it is useless.

Staff Nurse: You're right. It is important. I'll talk with the rest of the staff.

The student nurse was the assertive model for the charge nurse. This situation extends further, however, since the charge nurse found it difficult to approach the doctors regarding the handwashing issue, and the student nurse continued asserting herself. The following conversation ensued:

Assertive Student Nurse: Excuse me, I think it's important that everyone follow the hand-washing precautions when dealing with this patient.

Dr. Blue: Well. . . . *(his voice trails off)*

Assertive Student Nurse: I believe the reason this procedure was initiated is to protect the patient from being exposed unnecessarily to sources of infection. This can't be effective unless everyone takes part in it.

Dr. Blue: That's true. I'll wash my hands.

More often that not, it is difficult for nurses to be assertive with doctors. Doctors frequently ignore various nursing procedures while nurses stand quietly by. The above student nurse decided to assert herself.

Mr. Smith, a sixty-two-year-old man with throat cancer, had undergone a tracheostomy two years ago to halt the spread of cancer. He was in the hospital recently to await a carotid hemorrhage as the curative treatment had not stopped the cancer. His trach was to be suctioned two to three times per shift as well as cleaned once per shift. Despite the continued cancer growth, Mr. Smith was hanging on to life, conscious, and able to nod his head. He was receiving doses of morphine to decrease pain.

Doctor: Nurse, how is Mr. Smith tonight?

Assertive Nurse: He's doing fairly well but he's becoming weaker. He has increased secretions from his trach and we are suctioning him about three times a shift.

Doctor: Just don't suction him or clean his trach any more.

The example at this point relates to patient/consumer rights, the next section in this chapter. The patient not only has a right to determine whether he lives or is allowed to die but at the very least it is his right to be part of the decision if this is possible.

To move on—the patient was complaining of pain and was very restless.

Assertive Nurse: Would you increase Mr. Smith's dose of morphine?

Doctor: Yes, give him Morphine gr. ½.

Assertive Nurse: Would you write that in the order book?

Doctor: No, just give it.

Assertive Nurse: No, I want the order written before I give it because of the increased dosage.

While the nurse was being assertive on the patient's behalf, she was also being assertive for herself. The order written and signed by the physician indicated that he was aware of the increased dosage.

Between Nurse and Infant

In maternity a new mother who was learning to nurse her baby put on her light. The nurse answered the light and saw the infant crying and pulling away from the breast.

Mother (*while holding the baby loosely*): See, this baby does not want to nurse. Take her back to the nursery.

Assertive Nurse: It seems like that—try holding your baby a little more firmly near your body and stroke her cheek with your fingers. Here, I'll help you—sometimes babies need a little guidance when they first learn to nurse.

In this example, the nurse was being a patient advocate for the infant. Her actions helped the mother as well.

Between Nurse and Patient with Doctor

A seventeen-year-old woman patient who was in the first stages of labor was wincing and crying out. The doctor walked into the labor room to talk to her:

Doctor: You're not having any pain. Stop crying. I want to talk to you.

The patient continued to wince, cry out, and turn in bed. A male nurse came into the room, heard the doctor's words, and observing the patient's behavior, said to the physician:

Assertive Nurse *(to doctor)*: How do you know she is not having any pain?

Doctor : *(does not answer)*

Assertive Nurse *(to patient)*: It looks to me as if you are in beginning labor. Let me feel your abdomen. Yes, you are about two centimeters dilated and seem to be progressing in labor.

Between Nurse, Mother, and Patient

(On the phone.) Nurse: Your daughter has been in a car accident but she is alright. May we have your permission to sew her up? She received a small cut on her lip.

Mother: On her lip?

Nurse: Yes, it is pretty deep and needs to be sutured. Can we go ahead and do it?

Mother: No, I will come right over to the emergency room. I'm five minutes away.

Mother enters the emergency room five minutes later and finds her daughter crying.

Daughter: Mom, are you mad at me?

Mother: No, I am concerned about you. Why do you ask?

Daughter: Because the nurses and doctors are mad at you because you wouldn't give them permission to go ahead with my treatment.

Mother: That's right. I asked them not to suture your lip as I wanted a plastic surgeon to do it because it's on your face. I didn't know if the doctor on call was a plastic surgeon and I personally wanted to check that out.

Daughter: Oh!

Mother: I'm calling in a plastic surgeon now.

Two hours later, after meeting the physician, the mother makes a simple request—based on advocacy for her daughter. The following incident occurred:

Mother: My daughter has had a number of hospitalizations early in her life and has not understood what was happening to her. Please explain any procedure you do to her. This will ensure her cooperation.

Physician (*smiling and looking away*): Okay.

Mother: (*walked out of the emergency room during the suturing*).

Physician: (*Began fixing a syringe*)

Daughter: Is that novacaine?

Physician: (*Did not answer question but gave her the shot*). Oh! You want a quickie job, huh. I'll sew you up in 12 minutes. (*Began touching patient's mouth and lip.*)

Daughter: Ouch!

Physician: Oh, you want a quickie suture job—I'll sew you up quick.

Physician: He's seen my quickie jobs (*to the other physician in the room*).

Other Physician: You wouldn't want one of his quickie jobs— I've seen them.

Daughter: (*Quiet with tears in her eyes.*)

Physician: (*Began to sew up lip*) I can do quickie jobs if that's what you want. I think you would rather have the other kind.

At this point the two physicians began talking between themselves. Forty-five minutes later the mother walked in and heard her daughter ask:

Daughter: Are you done?

Physician: Yes.

Daughter: May I have something for pain?

Physician: We'll see how you do tonight.

The daughter was going home with her mother and it was now 11:30 P.M. (Six hours after the accident.)

Mother: Write a pain prescription for her.

Physician: O.K. (He did write the order). (The patient was sutured thoroughly).

Later this physician had his nurse call the mother to ask why the patient had not come to him to have the stitches removed. The mother repeated the above conversation. The nurse said, "Oh, he uses reverse psychology on adolescents." The mother explained how upsetting this entire event was to her daughter and that she understood explanations. The physician however did not give her this right nor respect. Clearly a patient advocate was needed in the emergency room to see that the mother's request to explain procedures was carried out by the physician.

TEACHING OTHERS TO SPEAK FOR THEMSELVES: TEACHING CONSUMERS' RIGHTS

The best person to speak for patient or consumer rights is the patient or consumer himself. Teaching patient/consumers they have the right to speak for themselves and be involved in health care decisions involving themselves and their bodies is high-level prevention and insures patient/consumer participation in health care issues. Standing up for one's rights and acting in one's best interest in addition are ways of maintaining feelings of self-control and self-management in the health care system, in contrast with feelings of powerlessness and depression that confront most patient/consumers who then behave as if they have no rights.

Consumers who assert themselves in asking for results of laboratory tests, X-rays, alternatives to surgery, asking questions regarding patients' rights, maternity benefits, natural child-birth, special diets, visiting hours, etc., initiate more openness and equality in interactions from nurses and other health professionals about health care.

The constitution speaks of equality for all and equal rights. At present there is no equality in the health care system and most people deny that they have rights even though they pay for care. Think about the last time you were a patient/consumer. Did you exercise the right to know what medicine and treatment you were obtaining and paying for? Was the health care delivered to you or did you go to the health care professional or institution? Were you given any preventive care or just treated? Were you satisfied with the communication skills between yourself and the physician, nurse, and institution? Were you made aware that a patient bill of rights existed? Were you given safe and competent care? Did you take an active role in decisions involving your health care and body?

As a nurse consumer of health care did you think about these kinds of questions? If so were you satisfied with the answers? Are you comfortable answering patient/consumers who ask similar questions?

Teaching assertion to the patient/consumer decreases the "elitism" surrounding medical and health care. Health care has been mystifying to the consumer who has been taught that knowledge of medical science is beyond his grasp. Patient/consumers have been rewarded for silence and not challenging or asking health professionals, particularly physicians, questions about illness, and hospitals about health care in general.

The evidence for this is the failure of several consumer-run health movements: for example, the popular health movement of 1830 to 1850, which wanted to eliminate the elitist system of doctor-craft in preference to self-care, and the community health movement proposed by President Kennedy and carried out by President Johnson in the early '60s. The women's movement is now presenting self-care (knowing your body, asking for what you want) options as an alternative system.

Nurses who can model assertive behavior in self-care areas will encourage patient/consumers to assert themselves. In addition, nurses who teach patient/consumers their rights are helping them to participate more equally and fully in their own health care.

Assertive behavior places more emphasis on prevention and wellness than on illness—the medical model that prevails at present in the health care system. Nurses' openness and willingness to discuss various questions consumers have regarding health care will distribute responsibility to the consumer and also motivate other nurses and physicians to keep up-to-date on knowledge. For example, funding to study women's diseases such as cancer of the cervix or breast is not always available because most of Congress is composed of males who, in addition to being older, are not affected themselves by the above diseases and often are not interested. Women consumers then must assert themselves by research and task forces to introduce bills on these issues. This behavior of choosing and giving public affirmation is assertion practiced in a sophisticated high-level wellness life stye.

Between Student Nurse and Patient

An adolescent boy was talking to a student nurse:

Patient: The doctors never tell me anything about what they're doing or planning for me.

Assertive Student Nurse: Have you asked them?

Patient: Yeah! But it seems like they don't hear me or don't care to answer.

Assertive Student Nurse: It's your right to get answers to your questions. Call your doctor and say, "I would like to know what your plans are for me. I want some answers so I will know what is happening to me and I can make plans." You have a right to know about your health and what the physician has in mind. This way you can agree or disagree. Patients have these rights as the American Hospital Association Patient Bill of Rights states.

Patient: Okay, I'll try.

The student nurse was encouraging the patient to take an active role in finding answers to his questions.

Between Nurse and Patient

In the psychiatric unit the following occurred. A patient was talking to a nurse.

Patient: I can't tell the doctor anything. I don't make sense when I get upset. You do it for me.

Assertive Nurse: What is it you wish to tell the doctor?

Patient: I just can't do it—no use talking about it.

Assertive Nurse: Try it—now what do you want to say?

Patient: Well, my wife will be at home alone this weekend and I . . . it's so silly.

Assertive Nurse: Go on.

Patient: I want to have an overnight pass so I can sleep with her. The children went to their grandparents and we would be alone.

Assertive Nurse: That sounds like a neat idea.

Patient: Yeah, but the doctor will never listen—you ask him for me.

Assertive Nurse: Wait a minute, what do you think he will say?

Patient: Oh, he'll look at the floor and say, "What do you want to do that for after she got so angry with you last Sunday?"

Assertive Nurse: Well, what would you say to that?

Patient: She was upset that the kids were there and her mother and she felt she had to take care of them so I left her alone. Later she said she was angry that I hadn't held her or told her I loved her and maybe I didn't care for her. I want to show her I love her.

Assertive Nurse: You certainly make sense when you practice what you want to say.

Patient: I did—didn't I, but it's a little embarrassing.

Assertive Nurse: Let's try it again—often the more you practice asking specifically for what your want, the real situation seems to go easier, particularly as you become more comfortable.

This nurse, by listening to the patient and gently insisting he try and put into words his request to the doctor, is teaching assertion to a consumer. In addition, the nurse is encouraging the patient to do behavior rehearsal so that when he confronts the physician he will be clear on what he wants to say.

If you, as a professional nurse, believe and practice assertive behavior, isn't it logical that patient/consumers whom you have taught to speak up for their health care rights might throw off some of their nonassertive dependency and gain in self-respect? Patient involvement in health care is as necessary as professional involvement. Doctors who make decisions and intrude upon emotional or physical aspects of others' bodies without their knowledge or understanding are utilizing extremely aggressive behavior. You, as a caring, professional nurse, have an obligation to help patients learn to speak out to obtain facts and participate in the decision-making process.

REFERENCES

Alberti, R. E., and Emmons, M. L. *Stand Up, Speak Out, Talk Back*. New York: Pocket Books, 1975.

American Hospital Association. *A Patient's Bill of Rights*. Chicago: 1973.

Cotler, S. B., and Guerra, J. J. *Assertive Training: A Humanistic-Behavioral Guide to Self-Dignity*. Champaign: Research Press, 1976.

Ehrenreich, B., and English, D. *Witches, Midwives, and Nurses: A History of Women Healers*. Old Westbury, N.Y.: The Feminist Press, 1973.

Herman, S. J. "Assertiveness: An Answer to Job Dissatisfaction for Nurses," in R. Alberti (ed.), *Assertiveness; Innovations, Applications and Issues*, San Luis Obispo, Calif.: Impact Publishing Co., 1977.

————. "Assertiveness Training," *The Hopkins Nurse*, Issue 4; January 1976.

————. "Differential Mutual Perceptions of Doctors and Nurses and Their Effects on Task Performance." Unpublished research paper presented at the Catholic University of America, Washington, D.C., 1972.

————. "Stereotypic Beliefs of Nurses." Paper presented at The Johns Hopkins University Assertion Training Workshop, February 1977.

Phelps, S., and Austin, N. *The Assertive Woman*, San Luis Obispo, Calif.: Impact Publishing Co., 1975.

Stein, Leonard. "The Doctor-Nurse Game," *American Journal of Nursing* (January 1968): 101–105.

6 Maintaining Assertive Skills: How To Keep Doing It

After reading and following the steps to assertion in this book, it is important to reinforce your newly learned skills. At this point most nurses are motivated and eager to practice the assertive skills over and over. This reinforces your new-found philosophy that assertive behavior brings about effective communication and good interpersonal relationships. In fact, only daily practice and use of assertive behavior skills will help you integrate them as a natural part of your behavior repertoire. Self-reinforcement and group reinforcement may encourage you to practice.

One of the best support systems available to increasing your use of assertive skills is self-reinforcement. Self-reinforcement is to praise and encourage, or to give things to yourself to increase the chances of repeating desirous behavior. In other words, by observing your behavior you can (1) exercise choice over behavior, (2) reinforce what you want to do internally as well as verbally, (3) make behavior lists, or (4) count to see how many times a desirous behavior is produced.

You may say, "Does it work?" Research in self-reinforcement as summarized by Kanfer (1970) demonstrates that it works. To give yourself a reward immediately after performing a desired behavior, such as after asking a physician to change his behavior, provides an immediate positive reinforcement of such desired behavior. This encourages you to repeat the behavior again when appropriate. The reward you choose can be material (money, a new dress, jewelry), internal (compliments, self-affirming thoughts), or an activity (going to the beach, the mountains, a play, or spending time talking with others). Whatever you choose, give it to yourself immediately after practicing the behavior. In other words, first work, then play or relax. Usually, the sooner the reward is given after performing the desired behavior, the quicker internal reinforcement begins to build.

REINFORCING AND MAINTAINING ASSERTIVENESS

Think Positive, Self-Affirming Thoughts Regarding the Particular Assertion

You decide to ask the Dean for permission to miss graduation exercises, though they are required. You have attended for the past five years, but have a chance to begin your trip to Europe earlier by not going. For self-reinforcement you might think the following or similar self-affirming thoughts:

> I have been a responsible, consistent faculty member and have been reliable in teaching, attending meetings, and being present at faculty-student functions. I very much want to leave a day earlier for Europe, as I can then spend an extra day going to the theater in London. I believe I can present my request in an appropriate manner and will be understood by the Dean. I will try anyway and if it is not accepted, I will be disappointed, but pleased that I tried.

Check out the particular assertion before and after by rereading either "Refusing Requests," "Making Requests," or "Asking for a Change in Behavior: Ideas to Keep in Mind" (Chapter 4).

Using the preceding example, you might reread "Making Requests: Ideas to Keep in Mind" and think to yourself, "I have a right to make a request and will do so by clearly and directly asking the Dean for permission to leave a day early for my vacation trip to Europe."

Use Verbal Self-Reinforcement

Say out loud, "After I practice making a request, this assertive behavior skill becomes easier, smoother, and feels more natural," or "I'm doing okay and I'm learning to assert myself." Hearing one's voice affirm an action is a self-reinforcer.

Keep an Assertive Record

Making a list of what behaviors you want to learn or of new areas in which you want to practice assertive skills will reinforce you to a more specific focus in your assertion. For example, making requests may be an assertive skill you already practice with your peers and colleagues; however, you rarely use this skill with authority figures. Identifying what assertions you want is most important for obtaining them.

Count Specific Assertions

Besides making the above list you can keep track of the number of times you actually practiced a behavior that day or week. For instance, to learn to assertively make requests count the number and kind of requests you make in a day. Then count the number made in a week. Now look to see if the requests you are making are the kind that you want to increase. If so, keep counting. If not, count only those you want to increase. Compare the number of requests you made each day with the previous day. Does this reinforce you?

Make Specific Assertive Contracts with Yourself for Difficult Areas and Develop Rewards for Each Step

Identify a personal plan of action. This entails identifying a skill and making a contract with yourself to practice the skill. Plan to and reward yourself as you practice. This reinforces your learning.

For example, at the annual Christmas hospital cocktail party and other similar group functions you find yourself listening instead of initiating conversations and then suddenly withdraw-

ing and leaving the party. You would rather initiate topics of
conversation and have others respond, or when you do listen
you want to then make verbal comments so that you are more
actively involved rather than becoming apathetic and withdrawing. This seems to happen more frequently in a group situation
rather than when talking with another person. At this point you
have identified behavior to learn and are ready to practice it by
taking a series of small graduated steps. The first step may be
(1) thinking of conversational topics you know about and are
interested in, (2) initiating a topic with others at a social
function, (3) making verbal responses to other comments that
show you have an interest in what you are saying and want to
add your ideas, or (4) using assertive skills such as giving and
getting information or self-disclosing, and putting these together in actual practice in group settings.

Before attending the next hospital cocktail party or social
function, decide to practice one or two steps of the above ideas.
For instance, after thinking of conversational examples, plan to
actively initiate a conversation. Next plan to reward yourself for
practicing this new behavior. The reward might be to take
yourself to a new play in town, read a book you've been putting
off, or spend time with friends. Reward yourself for sticking in
there and talking rather than leaving. Learn to reduce tension
beforehand by tightening and releasing leg muscles, hand
muscles, or arm muscles, or by standing instead of sitting all the
time. Remember, reshaping lifetime patterns of thinking, feeling, and behavior takes time and practice and patience.

As you practice, compliment yourself often by caring, positive
thinking that you are working to change behavior. This will
reward you for success, and with continual practice the new
behavior itself will bring rewards that will help you more
spontaneously maintain your new behavior.

Choose Assertive Individuals to Imitate or Model After

As you observe persons you particularly respect and admire,
notice what aspects of their behavior are attractive to you. Is it
their body posture, tone of voice, eye contact, or ability to

verbally express themselves? Try imitating the specific behavior that impresses you. Assertive trainers as well as effective head nurses, educators, nurse practitioners all can serve as effective assertive models, particularly if they personally demonstrate authentic, emotionally honest, and sincere behavior. Nurses who actively decide to imitate these assertive models are behaviorally reinforcing themselves.

Reread Chapter 4 or Related Chapters in This Book

Although most of you can help yourselves, some individuals in severe crisis situations may get more help working with a therapist. On the other hand, many of you, after learning basic assertive techniques, may discover yourself returning to nonassertiveness in response to anxiety. Do not hesitate to reread Chapter 4 and practice the exercises again. Although you don't have to assert yourself on each and every occasion, it is necessary to continue practicing the skills and consciously be aware of making assertive choices. Often nurses who in the past used mostly nonassertive responses may find themselves using aggressive ones. Don't be alarmed. This will change to assertion with more practice, and is considered very normal for women coming in touch with anger at many of the female sex role socializing conditioning processes that have kept them dependent on others. What happens is that suddenly nurses find they enjoy the freedom of saying what they think and feel and the release from anxiety that restrained them previously. This freedom changes to more self-control, and use of appropriate assertive behavior occurs as nurses are very concerned that they are not aggressive. There are some risks and negative consequences when first experiencing this free energy, so it is important to monitor your behavior as much as humanly possible. Relaxation exercises help channel this, as do speaking and behaving assertively.

Begin with Low-Risk Assertions and Build

Because self-reinforcement depends on the rewards gained and increasing self-esteem, it is important to begin with low-risk assertions. Asking strangers to loan you a match or for directions before asking your supervisor for a weekend off or your co-worker for a ride in her car pool are examples of building low- to high-risk assertions for most people. Asking a marital partner for a change in behavior might be an even higher risk, depending on the individual. In making these requests, consider if it is easier for you to ask of strangers, professional co-workers, or family members. Decide for yourself what situations or persons have low-risk consequences and which higher consequences. Then begin with low-risk situations, as success at this level will reinforce you to risk in more complex situations.

Group Support

Group support is an extremely valid way of obtaining reinforcement. In fact, most assertive training is taught in group situations, as much learning occurs from hearing about others' experiences and alternative solutions. You may want to combine the following ideas with self-reinforcement.

Follow-up Workshops

After reading this book, you may choose to attend a workshop. This, and the practice sessions, can help reinforce your self-learning. Watching trainers who model their individual style of assertion is one of the best ways you can learn assertiveness (Bandura, 1965; Eisler, Hersen, and Miller, 1973). In addition, having a group experience learning assertion not only reinforces you, but allows you to see many different styles of assertion from different group members. This will help you to integrate assertiveness into your personality. Learning assertion in groups can be fun as well as productive. You can ask for emphasis on role-playing actual work situations you may still be having trouble with or work on expanding other assertive skills.

Form Your Own Group

Another effective way to reinforce assertive skills is to form your own group in which members who have read this book (and specifically Chapter 4) decide to meet every other week for two months to role play and discuss implementing newly acquired assertion skills. At one institution five members met every other week at noontime, practiced assertive skills and behavior rehearsal, listened to one another's experiences, and supported one another in using assertive skills. Still another institution offered a room once a week where nurses could meet with a trainer to practice skills and discuss applications of assertion to nursing situations. Simply meeting together over lunch, talking assertively, and role enacting helped these nurses renew motivation, enthusiasm, and support for one another.

Reading and discussing within a group other books on assertion is another way to reinforce one's own assertiveness. Observing assertive behavior as it occurs on the television or movie screen are also ways of viewing assertive models or distinguishing the modes of assertion, nonassertion, and aggressiveness.

Join Other Relevant Groups

Joining a consciousness-raising group often broadens and helps one explore beliefs, attitudes, and values. Although change in behavior comes only from actual practice on certain behaviors (Lazarus, 1966), the issues in consciousness raising help women determine new priorities and open their eyes to alternate life styles. Almost every chapter of the National Organization for Women has consciousness-raising groups beginning or ongoing that need members. By contacting the National Organization for Women in your area, it is usually easy to join a new group. Many of the newest consciousness-raising groups are based on a ten-hour self-learning model (Perl and Abarbanell, 1976).

In these groups awareness evolves from sharing beliefs and attitudes toward issues regarding women and their sex role socialization process in general. As nurses you will personally, as well as professionally, find such topics as mothers and daughters, do women like women, female/male sex role characteristics, rape, women and economics, sexuality, feminism and lesbianism, or abortion extremely vital and very closely identified with nursing and the health care system. It takes time to sort out what you believe about these controversial issues. Until you are clear on what you believe, it's impossible to be assertive in those areas. Many of the above topics, besides being relevant for women in nursing, can help nurses learn to accept differences in one another, be assertive, be emotionally honest and sincere, learn to accept competence in themselves and other nurses, and collaborate to work with one another more effectively as a professional group.

Beginning or joining a value-clarification group is another alternative. These groups focus on identifying values that you consider highly important to your life style. Life goals and action plans are periodically reviewed to see if consistency between values and goals exist. More knowledge or emotional growth often stimulates a more thorough examination of values. To be more knowledgeable of your values helps reinforce your use of assertiveness.

Whether you use self-reinforcement or groups or both, maintaining assertive skills requires work until the behavior itself becomes comfortable and rewarding for you. At first, choose to work only in specific areas, and when you find your behavior reinforced spontaneously, choose other areas in which to practice.

REFERENCES

Bandura, A. "Behavioral Modification Through Modeling Procedures," in L. Krasner and L.P. Ullman (ed.), *Research in Behavior Modification.* New York: Holt, Rinehart & Winston, 1965, pp. 310–340.

Eisler, R.; Hersen, M.; and Miller, P. "Effects of Modeling on Components of Assertive Behavior," *Journal of Behavior Therapy and Experimental Psychiatry*, 4 (1973): 1–6.

Fensterheim, H. "Behavior Therapy: Assertive Training in Groups," in C.J. Sager and H. Kaplan (eds.), *Progress in Group and Family Therapy.* New York: Brunner/Mazel, 1972.

Kanfer, F.H. "Self-Regulation: Research, Issues, and Speculations," in C. Neuringer and J.L. Michael (eds.), *Behavior*

Modification in Clinical Psychology. New York: Appleton-Century-Crofts, 1970, pp. 178–220.

Lazarus, A. "Behavior Rehearsal Versus Nondirective Therapy Versus Advice in Affecting Behavior Change," *Behavior Research and Therapy,* 4 (1966): 209–212.

Perl, H. and Abarbanell, G. *Guidelines to Feminist Consciousness Raising.* Los Angeles, Ca.: 1835 South Bentley, 1976.

Uustal, D. "Searching for Values," *Image,* 9 (February 1977): 15–17.

7 Barriers to Nurses Becoming Assertive: What To Be Aware of and Overcome

You can become aware of assertive behavior and techniques in a relatively short period of time—six to ten hours. However, as you practice you will discover new ways to assert yourself, different alternatives, and new challenges in many varied situations. The health care system provides numerous situations for interactions with patients, physicians, or nurses that have the potential to be an assertive experience with positive consequences in terms of self-esteem. However, asserting yourself as a nurse requires not only patience and practice but awareness of and proceeding through some additional barriers. Because these barriers involve conflicting and paradoxical aspects this section may need to be read several times.

The barriers you as nurses need to be aware of and overcome are

The female sex role socialization process
The nursing socialization process
The unique nature of nursing
The belief system of nurses, which is perpetuated by nurses and the media

THE FEMALE SEX ROLE
SOCIALIZATION PROCESS

Since most nurses are women, we have been constrained by and inherited the early female sex role socialization messages. These have been effective barriers to our becoming assertive. We have noted many of these messages already. Specifically, these are that women are seen and see themselves as having a second-class status and are viewed stereotypically as passive, accommodating, submissive, helpless, unadventurous, dependent, emotional, and security oriented. (Millett, 1970; Broverman *et al.*, 1970) Traditionally, society sees women as existing or caring for others first and before thinking of their own needs. Because women were socialized to allow others to set goals for them rather than initiating their own, many lost sight of who they were or what they wanted as individuals from life for themselves. Many have settled for obtaining approval of others for accepting the female sex role socialization values. This means accepting specific messages of society to women: (1) Think of others first, even if you are hurt, angry, or tired, (2) be humble, never brag, tell others positive things about yourself, or be competent, (3) always listen, be understanding, compassionate, and never complain, (4) always find out what the other person is thinking or feeling—don't ever hurt others, and (5) be willing to give to others—don't expect financial reimbursement for services. These messages perpetuate compliant, submissive behavior and make learning to be assertive no easy accomplishment for women. In fact, to become assertive, women must choose some of the male sex role characteristic stereotypic behaviors, such as autonomy, independence, being active rather than reactive, adventurous, ambitious, and self-expressive (Broverman *et al.*, 1970). To choose these behaviors is often threatening, frustrating, and painful. Women making these choices often lose traditional support systems and because of such dependent attitudes and training confuse being feminine with being aggressive.

How to Overcome and Move On

For you as a nurse the first step is to become aware of yourself as a woman. Know your thoughts, feelings, and behaviors. Do you think and behave as others want you to or do you choose? Become aware of your thoughts on learning to be assertive. Do these encourage or discourage you to change behavior that stems from early female sex role socialization training? For example: the hospital unit you work on wants everyone to agree to resign to make a point. You do not agree, but no one else has mentioned believing this way. You do not verbalize that you disagree as you fear being different and making your co-workers angry with you. To not have their approval would be uncomfortable and awful. If this situation is familiar these thoughts are similar to all the traditional messages given to you and other women. Becoming aware of these thoughts will give you the opportunity to choose to change your thinking. (Refer to Chapter 3.) You might then make such self-enhancing self-statements as the following:

I think and feel differently from my colleagues. It's a new behavior for me to be different from others but I believe in not resigning and I am going to try it. Some of the nurses may be annoyed at me but I'll survive that. I care about myself and like myself and so don't need their approval for my self-worth. I will feel better about myself if I express my thoughts and hold to my views rather than take theirs.

By choosing to know your thoughts and changing self-defeating ones to specific rational thinking about a situation, you will allow yourself to experience positive feelings that will result in more assertive behavior for you. The catch is to listen to what you think, check it out with female sex role socialization messages, decide if your thoughts are self-enhancing to you as a person or self-defeating. If they are self-defeating, try changing them to more logical, objective ones. Notice your feelings then about yourself. Are they positive? If so, give yourself a compliment—"I can allow myself to think worthwhile self-enhancing thoughts. I like the resulting feelings." If you are still feeling guilty or angry, repeat the experience until your feelings are congruent with your more rational thoughts. As we saw in Chapter 3 this may involve strongly challenging your self-defeating thoughts.

The second step is to talk more assertively. To continue with the above example, you might say to your co-workers:

I understand you want everyone to quit to take a stand. However, I think and feel differently about the hospital unit situations. I choose to not resign.

Assertive comments like this may be difficult at first but are beginning ways to be you and do what you want. Practice like this helps you overcome behavior that was geared to others' approval rather than your own.

The third step may be joining a consciousness-raising group as mentioned in Chapter 6 or a rap group or reading additional books to sort out your feelings about women's issues and how you are affected.

THE NURSING SOCIALIZATION PROCESS

Another barrier that inhibits relating to self, patients, and co-workers effectively has been the nursing socialization process, which at times is similar to the female sex role socialization process. This process begins when students are accepted into a nursing education program and as they become indoctrinated into nursing look for effective role models such as educators and clinicians to follow. At this early stage students are confronted ever so subtly with conflicting, self-defeating, and at times paradoxical messages, which can be labeled the nursing socialization process. These messages are

1. To be independent as far as nursing knowledge and practice goes but to retain such values as sacrifice, humility, and "existing for others" (Phelps and Austin, 1975). Do not question or challenge issues that indicate your competence or knowledge.
2. To practice with a sound professional scientific knowledge base but not to become emotionally involved with patients, co-workers, or issues—maintain a professional role. Ignore conflict, deny your feelings and those of patients or co-workers—keep the environment calm and tension-free.
3. To be professional but not to expect equal professional financial reimbursement despite educational background and work performed.

4. To be an equal member of the health care team but not to participate in policy-making or decisions. Never compete with physicians in terms of patient care or show competence in other areas as we still need others to show us how.
5. To establish support systems for nursing but do not organize effectively for work tasks. Do what's best for everyone, don't say what you mean, don't let people know what you want, and mostly be silent and noncommittal.

Many of these conflicting messages were instigated by pioneers in nursing to obtain recognition and further the profession.

Let's look at how these messages have come about and how they can be recognized.

1. One early role model for obedience and service was demonstrated by Florence Nightingale. When Ms. Nightingale, with a group of nurses, demanded food and supplies to take to the Crimean War, and insisted upon proper shelter and sanitation facilities for the sick and wounded soldiers, her behavior demonstrated initiative, and independent thought and action.

Overwhelmed by her organizational skills and her staff of nurses, the doctors ignored Nightingale and her nurses when they arrived in Crimea. Then Nightingale refused to let her nurses begin to care for the thousands of sick and injured until the doctors gave an order. (Ehrenreich and English, 1973). The doctors were impressed and finally decided they could trust women who would follow their orders. Nightingale and her nurses began cleaning up the hospital and feeding the sick. This worked for nurses and has become a habit that has been perpetuated throughout the years. Later when Ms. Nightingale and her nurses spoke of their work they talked of the personal sacrifice they made to care for the injured and how dutifully they carried out their work. Perhaps in these early times nurses had to underplay their job to maintain their respectability in that society. Today Ms. Nightingale after an assertive training course might announce what satisfaction and honor she obtained from developing a plan to care for soldiers in wartime and to carry it out. No doubt today there would be a little financial reimbursement.

In hospital situations where initiative and independence is required for patient care and nurses do take twenty-four-hour care of patients, the nurse's ingrained belief in her subservient role is reinforced by physicians and other nurses and hinders her from fully accepting much authority commensurate with patient responsibilities. Behaviorally, nurses themselves perpetuate this by taking on other duties such as handing charts to physicians, or standing up and giving them their chair when they come into the nurses station, referring patient questions to physicians, or remaining silent after the doctor criticizes them unjustly in front of patients. Not that at times nurses may consciously choose to behave in the above manner as many do out of an assertive choice. Many nurses aren't aware, however, that they exhibit or have a choice to not exhibit this kind of behavior.

While the patient is of utmost importance in nursing, educators need to reinforce a progression of simple to complex learning, that is, know and care for yourself first, which enables you to help others know and care for themselves. It is important for you to as nurses to use "I" messages in speaking about yourselves as well as encouraging patients to use "I" messages when they explain what they want or how they are feeling. When nurses and patients use "I" messages this indicates their acceptance of responsibility for either patient care or their own care (in the patient's case). This helps both nurses and patients see one another as independent individuals. In addition this helps patients do more self-care. Unfortunately, much of education encourages nurses to speak with humility and subservience and often the following indirect messages are heard:

> Maybe if we did it this way
> Why not ask Dr. Smith
> Do you really believe that
> Why not check it out with her and then him
> and then decide
> What if we did it this way

rather that these:

> I believe it could work this way
> I'll ask Dr. Smith
> I'm interested to learn about
> I would like to do it this way

As we know, messages that use "I" statements tell who you are and reinforce your thoughts and ideas. This helps develop your identity and authenticity as a person. Of course, communicating this directly is risky, since you can't know if others will agree before you make a statement. In addition, using "I" statements tells others that you believe in yourself and think you are equal to others. It does not indicate humility or sacrifice; therefore, nurses who try to accept the conflicting message "be independent but don't be" become confused and often end up with low morale and dissatisfied with nursing (Herman, 1977).

2. Nurses have been involved in caring for patients on intimate physical levels since the inception of the profession. They closely work with patients after surgery, accidents, in long-term illnesses, and in rehabilitation. Despite this intimate physical nurturing and caring nurses are not to become involved emotionally with patients. In addition there are covert messages for nurses not to speak directly with one another or with physicians. Particularly, nurses are taught by educators and service role models not to be direct with physicians in a patient's presence, although physicians may do so with nurses.

This is evident in how nurses limit what they say in terms of refusing requests, asking for change in behavior, giving information, or handling criticism. When asked, nurses say they practice this behavior of withholding information for fear of not being perceived as competent to give patient care, fear of hurting patient feelings when they are ill, fear of being criticized by either their supervisors or physician, and fear of making the physicians or their colleagues angry with them. These fears perpetuate traditional values of servitude and dependence, which do not reinforce the nurse's respect for herself or reinforce autonomous behavior.

Other nurses believe that stating their thoughts or feelings directly will provide the option for patients or staff to label them as aggressive. Since aggressive behavior is incongruent with nurturance and caring, to be labeled as such even though it may not be true would present an insurmountable conflict to nurses who are taught to be considerate of others at all times. In fact, such nurses burden themselves with guilt that they are not "good nurses" if they do not appear or are not always nurturant and caring twenty-four hours a day to anyone no matter what the circumstance.

These fears or beliefs are incompatible with the patient advocate role. On the one hand, the nurse is taught to utilize expert communication skills and constantly provide clarity while, on the other, at the same time no feelings or emotions are supposed to be part of the communication. Consequently, when three or more people, such as patient, nurse, and physician, are involved in a communication system that is not direct and feelings are mostly denied, confusion is often the result. To complicate issues the nurses often talk to one another about the injustice done to the patient or the physician rather than directly to the person involved. Emotions are ventilated but to the wrong person. When this nonassertive behavior is practiced high anxiety and low self-esteem are the result for all participants in the interaction.

Nonassertive behavior is perpetuated by nurses keeping themselves busy, or allowing themselves to be kept so busy taking care of patients, that a habit of ignoring one's rights becomes established. It often becomes a top priority for nurses to complete all their work plus care for any additional crises that arise before thinking of themselves as nurses. Nurses trained to express themselves through meeting others' needs and caring for others rarely consider taking time to consider themselves or their human rights as they are working. When a habit of not thinking about yourself until your work is completed is repeated over and over a process of self-denial is reinforced. This leads to isolation from thoughts, feelings, opinions, and beliefs, and interferes with the nurse's functioning in an autonomous manner. Not being able to comply with these conflicting messages, nurses often feel guilty. What is even more confusing or paradoxical is when students discover that it is not only all right but nurses are covertly encouraged to also provide the "powerful" physicians with intellectual and emotional support. They are not to challenge or confront physician's decisions despite data they may have observed or collected. These conflicting covert messages are received by nursing students as they observe the behavior of nurse educators and clinicians. Emotionally confused, many nurses begin relating indirectly when conflicts occur, establishing a habit of not relating with authentic thoughts and feelings and thus unknowingly beginning to deny themselves basic human rights.

Nurses who do integrate the above mixed values manage to "not rock the boat" but at personal costs to themselves, as reflected in headaches, anxiety, and low self-esteem. Although this is congruent with the subservient behavior expected of nurses because of female sex role socialization, many nurses aren't aware that nursing socialization reinforces these conflicts. This behavior prevents nurses from being decisive, therapeutic role models who could help nurse colleagues as well as patients learn to assert their rights and autonomy in regard to conflicts regarding decisions concerning health problems.

3.   Nurses are taught that helping others is a service and a pleasure. While this is true in most aspects, after a nurse completes her education why is it that she doesn't obtain financial rewards commensurate with other professionals at the same educational level or as other people who have no educational training? Only professional aspects of nursing are discussed, not financial rewards. Nurses in private practice often offer their services at lower fees to clients or because of lack of self-esteem regarding their nursing competence. Why? Underlying this may be the myth that giving quality care at a lower fee may be virtuous or show humility and therefore be acceptable to other nurse or health care colleagues. Our economic system is a determinant of how we live. Nurse practitioners who must rely on one income and may be supporting a family often cannot afford to stay in nursing.

Nurse consultants are often expected to do extra work and are paid less than other consultants. Often nurse consultants work with no contract. Staff nurses work overtime or educators plan or attend workshops on vacations while not being financially reimbursed. The differentiation of pay between diploma and baccalaureate nurses is minimal, although between baccalaureate and master's level nurses there is more difference, though not comparable to other professionals with master's degrees.

4.   Nurses are educated to believe they are equal members of the health care team but at the same time they ask if they can do health teaching, if their ideas are all right, if they should talk

with the parents on pediatrics wards when asked health questions about their hospitalized children, and rarely are they leaders or administrators of health care centers, hospitals, clinics, or school health programs.

A group of nurses in two large hospitals in the East were very upset over similar incidents. They asked the physicians about the lack of care of long-term chronic children who were hospitalized and received no answer. The nurses asked physicians for medication orders and were told "don't bother me." The nurses persisted and the physician in charge in one hospital said, "The best thing you girls can do is follow our orders." The physician in the other said, "Let's get it straight, physicians are in charge here—we'll take care of the situations." Neither situation improved and the nurses did what they could without interfering or going to anyone else, probably because of the paradoxical socialization message "Be independent but be silent and subservient." These nurses stated, "We would have been aggressive to do anything else." The head nurses and supervisors also acquiesced.

The health team is often not composed of nurses and physicians but of social workers or psychologists, occupational therapists, or various technicians. Nurses have long experienced being taught by physicians. This practice now has mostly become antiquated, except in the most traditional of health care institutions. However, psychologists are often hired to teach nurses interpersonal skills or to help plan programs for nurses. Nurses are educated and prepared to plan programs as well but the myth among nurses is that we still need help—we aren't capable enough yet. Let's bring someone else in. When are we going to be competent? Is there a secret test some secret person will give nurses?

5. Nursing education and service consistently speak about the necessity for support systems for themselves in regard to decision making or any change that is to be implemented. However, it is never communicated what a support system is or how to establish one that doesn't fall apart. Support systems that exist and grow do so because of common beliefs and emotional investments of the nurses involved. Nurses who were trained not to commit themselves personally or emotionally to patients

find it difficult to do this with one another. Lacking professional role models in both education and service who autonomously stand behind issues, students are unable to implement such ideas. For example, after assertive training nurses often ask who will support them to be assertive. This request is reasonable in some aspects as nurses who are honest with one another can support one another. However, nurses, who have not experienced emotionally honest support systems before, but who have heard and experienced lip service regarding such support, remain confused as to what is going on or what is real support. Too many still believe it is catastrophic not to have lip service support of one another even though the other person doesn't really agree with you. That is not really support. For instance, after a two-hour assertiveness presentation by the author to over one hundred nurses, the nursing director in summary said, "Now that you have learned some assertiveness don't use it here." The participants laughed but the issue remained—we were given assertiveness through the inservice department and yet our director says don't use it here. The question these nurses were confronted covertly with was will we be supported if we try assertiveness? This obsessive need to always be supported can be identified in many nursing programs. Are most nurses so weak they cannot make statements unless someone agrees?

In many support systems covert rules exist. One is that everyone must have a say in decision making but that nurses must say what will please others. If everyone has a part in decision making few decisions are made and it's hard to tell who is accountable. To say what will only please others wastes endless amounts of time. Besides, no authentic feedback or reinforcement can be given or received if nurses are playing a perpetual guessing game of reading the expressions of others, if they seldom take stands, make bland statements, are perennially asking questions instead of making positive declarations, and generally are indecisive. While often this is done with the motivation of not hurting anyone's feelings, the overall effect is that individuals hide their feelings and massive ambiguity, vagueness, and indecisiveness results. These patterns continue in groups and promote an ongoing cycle of self-defeating or self-fulfilling unproductive behavior. Nurses who have been taught to say only what they believe others want to hear rather than what they themselves think or feel can easily lose their identity. After practicing this indirect behavior for years and being reinforced, it is impossible to know what you think or feel.

While it is true that women generally have not been listened to or been supported by society for what they think (Millett, 1970), in other professions such as law, business, or medicine women do seem to speak out more independently to define their competencies as professionals. Nurses need to practice speaking to their competencies and to controversal issues, taking independent action in work situations, and practicing listening to one another and giving authentic emotional support. Unless this happens nurses will remain dependent on others to make decisions and choices and this behavior resembles the traditional all-nurturing housewife or mother figure rather than a professional. Professionals can think independently, agree and disagree with one another, but still work together.

How to Overcome and Move On

Becoming aware of oneself and of the existence of these conflicts is a first and necessary step. Know what you think and feel about yourself as a person in different situations. Do you make choices and decisions to establish your priorities? Do you choose to use assertive skills in the health care system or only in social situations? Most important is to decide if you want to be unconflicted, that is, be fairly independent, practice as a professional without concealing emotions with patients and others, expect financial recompense for your work, act as an equal member of the health care team, and be authentic in groups to encourage the development of real support systems. In other words, will you demonstrate independence, self-power, autonomy, or subservience, sacrifice, and humility? You cannot do both. After you make the decision, hopefully for independence, begin speaking, carrying your body, and behaving in the same way. Take small risks at first and build until people on your unit become used to your assertive manner. Offer to talk to them about being assertive, tell them you are trying to make requests in a new way, or suggest workshop or reading materials.

Make decisions to listen to your thoughts in relation to your fears. What are these thoughts? When you find yourself thinking "I don't know much, I can't stand alone; I must not have enough data (when you listened exactly to what the patient said), begin to challenge with self-affirming thoughts. "I do know nursing content although I may not have all the answers all the time," "I can speak up for what I believe; however, every now and then it is a help to discuss the issue with a colleague," or "I did listen to what the patient said and arrived at a decision. The decision is a hard one; however, it is based on the actual data."

Take time to make a list of the number of occasions you speak in "I" messages during a day. If you make less than ten, actively practice making more.

Make a list of the number of times you withhold information. Is this a conscious choice? What are the particular situations? What are your fears? Do you do this more with peers, physicians, or patients? Do you share this information with others who aren't involved later in hopes they will support you? Identify examples and your thoughts regarding the examples.

Set aside time just for you once or twice a day. When is it? What will you give yourself as a reward for having special time to yourself?

Make a list of issues at work that you feel strongly about. Which ones have you taken stands on? Do you try to find out others' views and persuade them to your way of thinking?

How do you reinforce yourself for using assertive behavior? What rewards do you give yourself?

THE UNIQUE NATURE OF NURSING

While a hospital admits people who are ill, the major twenty-four-hour responsibility for patient care is carried by the nursing service. Although nursing has the responsibility, the major authority for giving patient care rests with the physician. This splitting of responsibility and authority for a job not only promotes powerlessness, ambiguity, and tension, but limits nurses' control over patient care. This reinforces the helplessness and dependence nurses feel, and adds to the confusion as to whom they are responsible—the patient, the physician, both, or the institution. An example of this splitting of responsibility from authority was given in Chapter 4. This incident occurred in a maternity ward in which the patient told the nurse she had taken natural childbirth courses and that the breathing helped her with labor. A few minutes later a doctor walked in and ordered a spinal. It was done and the nurse said nothing to the physician about the previous conversation nor did the patient. Nor did the doctor ask the patient. After the spinal the patient asked if the procedure would interfere with her having the baby born naturally.

Basically, the nurse by her silence demonstrated nonassertive and aggressive behavior by discounting what the patient had said previously. The nurse did not question the doctor's authority but colluded with him, giving up previously acknowledged responsibility in regard to the patient's communication.

This situation is an example of mythically evaluating human beings on scales in which some persons are seen as "better" than others (see Chapter 2). Acting as if some people have more or less value than others is not only unrealistic in the nursing profession but complicates the main task—that of patient care. Individuals who occupy the roles of patient, nurse, administrator, and physician are human beings. This is not to say that human beings do not occupy hierarchical roles in a bureaucratic system, such as a hospital, which carry differing kinds of authority, or that the authority of a supervisor in the system does not carry power and weight. What is of more value and equal importance is that nurses, as individual human beings, have their own authority and right to be respected, much as the larger hierarchical bureaucracy has a right to be respected. In other words, individuals have as much right to be heard as does the institution. Nurses do not believe they have a right to be heard and at times these rights seem more complicated in a hospital service institution, which takes care of living and dying persons, because of the general pervasive constraints of uncertainty and anxiety surrounding illness. This is substantiated in the health care systems by the myth that silence is golden in heavily-laden emotional situations. Silence does not only not help patients who are faced with uncertainties that require decisions, but it does not help the staff, nurses, doctors, and administrators who work to resolve these uncertainties. The combined emotional and intellectual complexity for nurses of working in a health setting fraught with anxiety because of life-threatening situations and death occurrences can only promote conflict, thus making assertive communication and mutual respect between people even more important.

The women's movement has reinforced nurses in regard to overcoming some of these nursing socialization process messages but clearly many internal conflicts still exist.

How to Overcome and Move On

Becoming aware and identifying these conflicting messages will help you choose what behavior you wish to exhibit. Being able to verbally assert yourself will enable you to prevent some of the conflicts before they arise. People cannot read minds. You must speak out.

Openly discussing these conflicts when they arise with other nurses will help in terms of group awareness, particularly if components of these conflicts are subtle.

Know nursing theory and clinical content so that you can speak up when paradoxical messages occur in emotional situations which involve head nurses, physicians, patients, administrators, and yourself. Oftentimes, speaking the obvious reduces anxiety in a tense situation. If you can't think of what to say, just say "It is certainly tense here. Let's see how we can reduce the tension."

When applying for jobs be aware of the conflicting messages and ask for job descriptions. Make sure the description is written and includes what you are expected to do, how much you will be paid, the extent of your authority and responsibility, and your title. Ask yourself if this is what you want.

Find out the lines of authority both formal and informal as they exist in the institution where you will be working by talking to other employed nurses. Will you be satisfied with your position?

In giving patient care, decide whether you are comfortable involving patients in their own care. If so do health teaching and encourage patients to make decisions that affect their health care and bodies. Act as a listening person and encourage patients to work out their conflicts. Talk this over with the staff and encourage others to help patients be involved in their health care.

The most important issue is to resolve your conflicts so that you can be free to decide a plan of action. This will allow you to exercise your interpersonal rights and help the patients or consumers exercise theirs. The conflicts that we have illustrated if not noticed and resolved can be professionally and personally devastating to nurses. Evidence of this is seen in the research quoted in Chapter 1 on the morale of nurses, high job turnover, and job dissatisfaction. This was found because of lack of personal satisfaction and nurses denying they have a right to interpersonal satisfaction. The implication is that professionals who deny one another human rights can hardly allow the patient or consumer rights.

THE BELIEF SYSTEM OF NURSES PERPETUATED BY NURSES AND THE MEDIA

Recent research data at assertiveness workshops oriented toward nursing documents that many nurses hold more irrational than rational beliefs about themselves, colleagues, and physicians (Herman, 1977). Becoming aware of these beliefs and changing them to rational ones will make it easier for nurses to practice assertive behavior skills and support one another in doing so.

The following are beliefs that nurses identified in a number of workshops out of which much of the data for this book came about. The beliefs staff nurses have regarding superiors— administrators, head nurses, and supervisors of nurses—are:

We do all the work.

They never see me as an individual and don't know procedures.

I know more about how the patients are and what they are doing than supervisors.

I'm the real nurse—supervisors are busy shuffling papers.

I carry too heavy a work load.

They do not see us as people and are manipulating.

They are quick to criticize, never give positive acknowledgement, not involved in planning patient care, give unfair assignments, show partiality, and never have to work weekends.

As a resourceful person
Can't question
Threat
Good administrator
Doesn't listen
Helper
Too much to do
Too objective

The following are what nurse administrators, supervisors, and head nurses believe about staff nurses:

Staff nurses don't understand the large job and responsibilities we have, their job descriptions, and don't take responsibility for disciplining their own team and for patient care and self-development.
Don't take advice or counseling.
They are necessary to carry out orders but too assertive.
They dump on us, are a threat, and are limited as people.
Staff nurses take no initiative, are insignificant, and are as a number.
As individuals, they do not challenge.

The following are the beliefs nurses, educators, students, clinicians, administrators, and staff have of doctors:

They're not appreciative
Moody
Infallible
Dedicated
Mercenary
Mind readers and male chauvinist pigs
Doctors are godlike, afraid to make mistakes, and if they do, do not admit to mistakes.
They are easily threatened.

The following are beliefs nurses, educators, students, clinicians, administrators, and staff have about how M.D.s perceive them:

We are handmaidens and they are unwilling to let us grow; faceless, insignificant, lower class, mind readers, less intelligent, subservient, sex objects, lackeys, and team members.

We think doctors believe we are women who should nurture them.

We think doctors believe we show favoritism, are a bother, and nag.

The following are the beliefs nurse administrators and educators have about doctors:

They are strong, protect each other, and have high status.

They make desirable husbands.

They are treated as godlike, regardless of illegible handwriting and bad personal relations skills.

They are knowledgeable but do not think nurses have knowledge.

They sabotage nurses and work from a power base.

They use nurses to clean up messes they leave.

They are reductive, domineering, insensitive, superior, and opinionated to nurses.

Nurse practitioners believe staff nurses are

Given scut work
Underutilized and used as escorts to rooms
Assistant to M.D.
Answer phone
Traffic control
Passive-aggressive
Hostile
Nonassertive
Give negative reinforcement for assertive behavior, nurses and M.D.
Concert power struggles
Handmaid to M.D.
Content with role
Discontent with role as
Nurse-Doctor game
Angry—internalize

Nurse practitioners believe staff nurses perceive them as

Equal but having different duties
Wish to have practitioner skills themselves
Don't know what a practitioner is
Gutsy
Leery of practitioner knowledge
Don't trust
We have similar knowledge
Frustrated M.D.
Glorified M.D. assistants
Resent practitioner skills
Threatens us

Nurse practitioners believe doctors perceive nurse practitioners as

Grateful
Part of team
Helped or shared responsibility
As added responsibility
Bothersome, what do you do?
Noncommittal

Nurse practitioners believe doctors are

Ultimate decision-makers
Incapable of admitting error
Resourceful persons
Set in ways
Experienced
Learned
Confident
Powerful
Influential
Lacking in humility

Student nurses believe doctors are

Power figures that need to feel that they do indeed have power
Open to manipulation
Egotistical
Public glorified
Upper-class
Self-serving
Not whole people—emotionally immature
Expediency getting
Arrogant
Omnipotent
Unethical/ethical
Stubborn
Authoritarian
Defensive
Witty
Career-minded
Aggressive
Money wasteful
Competent?
Foreign
Scientific
Efficient
Limited in scope or interest, narrow-minded
Insecure

Student nurses believe doctors perceive them as

A member of the team
A source of valuable information about a patient
A consultant
A patient advocate
A counselor able to relate as a person
Inferior to, less competent, knowledgeable, intellectual than themselves
Questioning authority and interfering
Subservient
Competition in the health field

Student nurses believe head nurses or faculty and supervisors are

Head Nurses
Mostly women
Generally older
Don't do bedside nursing
Fat "battle axes" "big frame"
Frowning a lot
Don't know meaning of
    specific nursing
    procedures
Task oriented—which side
    gets clean sheets
Complain about doctors noise
    up to them at the same time.
Tend to mother staff nurses
    as "My girls"
Alienated from health nurses
60 year old gray hair broad
    180 lbs, 5'9"
Brusk, strong, husky women
Domineering
Not married or with a
    husband 5'2"
Skinny and nervous
Rigid
Unhappy
Prone to rules
Stratified attitude
Efficient, cold, bright, warm,
    attractive open and verbal,
    cool

Faculty
Too idealistic
Young, white
Inconsistent in teaching and
practice
Nice (genuinely) people
All nurses
All women
Research oriented
Not classroom oriented
Not very good speakers

Student nurses believe head nurses, supervisors, and faculty perceive student nurses as

Threats to routine care on the floor
Manpower, particularly in relation to doing that which
staff people aren't particularly interested in doing
Idealistic, naïve

Role models for staff (showing staff how to do care plans)
More hindrance than help
Not adequately prepared, trained
Certain areas, student nurses can be helpful to patient
Student nurses don't know enough about what they talk
about and they are there to learn, not contribute.

How to Overcome and Move on

Since maintaining a positive belief system is congruent with asserting yourself (Lange and Jakubowski, 1976), nurses might engage in more assertive behavior by working to increase their positive beliefs. Developing basic beliefs (1) "that, assertion rather than manipulation, submission, or hostility enriches life and ultimately leads to more satisfying personal relationships with people and (2) everyone is entitled to act assertively and to express honest thoughts, feelings, and beliefs" (Lange and Jakubowski, 1976) would seem to benefit nurses.

There are several ways to do this.

Practice the rational emotive approach (refer to Chapter 3) to become aware of your thoughts in regard to events. Decide which are rational and which irrational.

Reread the ten irrational ideas. Read particularly the one that says when other people behave unfairly they should be severely put down. Nurses often feel they are treated unfairly and become angry when they or patients have been treated unfairly. To continue believing it is terrible and catastrophic and that the person who treats them this way should be severely punished only uses up one's energy. It will be more productive to dispute this irrational idea by using self-statements—"The world isn't fair," or "Why should the world be fair?" or "I don't like to be treated unfairly, how can I reverse the situation?" These rational self-statements help reduce your anxiety so that you can decide how to proceed. Self-defeating beliefs that things ought to or must be or should be different are based on fantasy. A more realistic belief might be that things would be better if they were different. How can I make them different?

Learn to confront irrational beliefs. When you develop challenges ask yourself the following questions: "Is this self-statement 100 percent true?" "Am I generalizing?" "What do I fear will happen?" "Is this reasonable?" "If this happened, would it be a catastrophe?" "Could I handle it?" Remember, generalized thoughts or beliefs perpetuate emotional dishonesty and low self-esteem. This happens on both an individual and on a professional level. Challenging or confronting these thoughts and beliefs increases one's assertive thinking; therefore, behavior and beliefs help you gain self-control. The following are examples of how to confront some of the irrational beliefs nurses have identified:

Event: As nurse educators and administrators, what do you believe doctors believe about you?

Irrational belief: Nurse educators and administrators believe doctors think they are intellectually inferior.

Questions to ask yourself: "Have nurse educators and administrators asked all doctors if they believe this?" "Is it possible some doctors consider nurses intellectually equal?" "If doctors should think nurses are inferior intellectually to them what will happen?" "Can you handle it if doctors think you are inferior to them?"

Rational belief: Nurse educators and administrators may confront the above irrational belief by saying to themselves "I think some doctors may believe nurse educators and administrators are intellectually inferior. I think others do not. I am not intellectually inferior as a person or as a nurse. I do not know medicine as physicians do. If some doctors do think I am inferior that is their option. I do not have to be controlled by what others think."

This type of rational confrontation of one's thoughts and beliefs allows nurses to change irrational thoughts and in turn increases self-worth and decreases anxiety.

Here is another example:

Event: As nurses what do you believe about doctors?

Irrational belief: Nurses, educators, students, clinicians, staff believe doctors are godlike.

Questions to ask yourself: "What is it about doctors that resembles a god?" "What do I fear that I need to see doctors as godlike?" "What will happen if I should believe doctors are people like everyone else?" "What other ideas do I have about sickness or medicine that are fearful?"

Rational belief: "Doctors are not gods and have human

qualities, some of which are positive and some negative. Some doctors may act as if they are gods but I don't have to believe it is so. If I believe doctors are people, then I can confront them as people who have the right to express thoughts, feelings, beliefs, and opinions as I have the right to express myself."

If you continue to confront these beliefs you will find more positive ways of interacting with people and you will be behaving in an assertive manner.

Exercise personal and interpersonal rights (Chapter 2). This is easier when you decide to think more rationally. Usually, the reason people do not accept their personal rights is they do not believe they are entitled to them. Watching how you think and identifying your beliefs can help you fully exercise your personal rights.

The common factor in the barriers identified is the inability to communicate thoughts, opinions, and feelings in a personally satisfying and effective manner (Herman, 1977).

Begin and get involved in a consciousness-raising group for nurses. Explore issues of sexism and sexism in nursing and the health care arena. How can you eliminate this? Get to know other nurses as women outside of a professional role and begin to develop emotionally honest support systems. This may be the first time you have had real support. Traditionally, women have not had one another's support and instead have been set against one another—"who needs to work for her?" "I'd rather work for a male boss any day." These messages only perpetuate the notion that women (nurses) have no worth and do not help nursing but rather support the traditional female sex role socialization process.

Confront the media: for example, a professional nursing journal that on its front cover publishes a cartoon of an obese nurse carrying a hypodermic syringe chasing a male patient or within the journal prints drug ads that show a nurse combing a patient's hair. Discuss this stereotyping of nurse images with other nurses and your friends. Notice the television serials that show nurses in Doctor Welby type programs. Do they represent us as professionals? Numerous films such as *M.A.S.H.* or *One Flew Over the Cuckoo's Nest* also portray nurses as sex objects or undesirous characters in general and perpetuate many of society's irrational ideas about nurses. Discuss these and what alternative nurse models or images you would like to have society see on television or in movies.

REFERENCES

Ehrenreich, B., and English, D. *Witches, Midwives, and Nurses: A History of Women Healers*. Old Westbury, N.Y.: The Feminist Press, 1973.

Millett, Kate. *Sexual Politics*. New York: Doubleday & Co., 1970.

Broverman, I.D. *et al.* "Sex Role Stereotypes and Clinical Judgements of Mental Health," *Journal of Consulting and Clinical Psychology*, Vol. 54, 1970.

Herman, S.J. "Assertiveness: An Answer to Job Dissatisfaction for Nurses," In B. Alberti (ed.), *Assertiveness: Innovations, Applications, Issues*. San Luis Obispo, Calif.: Impact Publishers, 1977.

————. "Differential Mutual Perceptions of Doctors and Nurses and Their Effects on Task Performance." Unpublished research paper presented at The Catholic University of America, Washington, D.C., 1972.

————. "Stereotypic Beliefs of Nurses." Paper presented at the Johns Hopkins University Assertion Training Workshop, February 1977.

Lange, A.J., and Jakubowski, P. *Responsible Assertive Behavior: Cognitive/Behavioral Procedures for Trainers*. Champaign, Ill.: Research Press, 1976.

Phelps, S., and Austin, N. *The Assertive Woman*. San Luis Obispo, Calif.: Impact Publishers, 1975.

8 A Look to the Future: Benefits of Assertiveness Training For Nurses

YOU CAN USE YOUR NEW SKILLS

In looking ahead, assertive skills can be of benefit to nurses in many ways. One very important benefit is to free us from anxiety and subservient behavior, which has plagued us since the inception of nursing. We as assertive nurses, by speaking clearly, concisely, and sincerely, become anxiety free. This gives us the freedom to consciously choose when to assert ourselves and when not to assert ourselves. This appropriate and flexible use of assertive skills allows your own style of assertion where you think it is appropriate. Times when you may choose not to assert yourself may be when the other person knows nothing about assertive behavior, when a passive response might be more helpful, when someone is undergoing severe emotional or physical stress, or when you encounter an angry, hostile person.

Other areas in which assertiveness benefits nurses are in job hunting, creating jobs, increasing one's personal effectiveness, increasing one's ability to work with nurses, increasing one's ability to work as a colleague with physicians, teaching patients to assert themselves, and as change agents in general. You will notice that as you read you will come up with other ways of possible future benefits in applying assertiveness.

Job Hunting

Assertiveness training is a valuable asset for any nurse who is job hunting. Looking for a job requires assertion skills in taking the initiative and making requests in the areas of interviews, filling out application blanks, having an up-to-date resume, talking to people, and making appointments. This can be a time-consuming process and very frustrating. Remember, you have the right to ask questions about working hours, salary, fringe benefits, promotion, and what is expected of you at work. The other person has the right to refuse to answer. However, some questions may require definite answers and you may consider working elsewhere if no answers or unsatisfactory answers are forthcoming.

You may have many interviews. In addition, you may have to talk to only one person at a time or to a group of five or six. In any case, be as relaxed as possible. You may want to practice some of the breathing or relaxation exercises before the interviews. It is helpful also to rehearse answers to any questions that might require a concentrated effort to include pertinent facts you want to get across.

During the interview, you will want to practice direct and appropriate eye contact, an erect body posture, a firm but pleasant voice, as well as responding in a direct, genuine way to questions or information about which you are asked. Initiating questions, shaking hands with the interviewers, negotiating salary, and clarifying any issues that arise all require assertion. You might also observe if your prospective employer and other interviewers are assertive in manner. To accept a position after being interviewed by people who are generally nonassertive may not be in your best interest. Be alert and observe.

Creating Jobs

Because the need for health care is so great, nurses now but even more so in the future will have the opportunities to create their jobs. This has been seen in isolated areas on Indian reservations, in the mountain and hill country, in hospitals where a nurse is needed to coordinate or provide a liaison, in clinics where nurses administrate and perform practitioner duties, in home deliveries of infants, in health teaching agencies, and in private practice. As more nurses develop assertive behavior and challenge conventional roles for nurses, other financially productive jobs will appear on the market. Nurses are tired of being silent and subservient when they possess knowledge and competent skills that are marketable in many new, unique ways to provide quality care for others.

To Help You Work Effectively

After you have found or created the job—whether it is in a hospital clinic, health center, industrial or educational institution—it is beneficial to use assertive skills to acquaint yourself with others, learn who your colleagues and supervisors are who will help you get the job done, and be able to work out any conflicts that arise when more than one nurse is working. It may be important not to overextend yourself, to find additional information about specific aspects of the job, to negotiate further working hours, or to extend caring assertions to the staff with whom you will be working. Remember your rights and also that others have rights. When first beginning a new job many frustrations may occur. It is important to use your assertive skills to overcome low frustration tolerance. This will improve self-control and increase feelings of self-worth. It will make the transition to to a new job easier. View your use of assertion as a gift to yourself.

Working with Other Nurses

As nursing students you learned the benefits of sharing with others in the course ideas about nursing and problems that occurred in the classroom and clinic. Nursing education in a sense has a built-in support system if utilized in an assertive way. In hospitals and educational and industrial institutions individual nurses can build this kind of support system. At times the system does not support genuine communicative relationships or it perpetuates the finding of scapegoats. In other words when it creates crises and blaming it on one nurse becomes a pattern, this leaves you wondering if you will be elected the next time. This not only increases low self-esteem for the nurses, but allows a situation that requires a lot of energy to analyze and combat. Some systems have a pattern of setting nurses against nurses. In these instances it is best to quit and to look for another job. In others, individual nurses can create satisfactory relationships within the system. This occurs where nurses remind themselves of their basic interpersonal rights, give one another emotional support and honest feedback, are available for one another, and share in stressful situations. Oftentimes, unions are the answer. Grievances must be satisfactorily dealt with so that nurses can continue to give approval and positive reinforcement to one another. This combats the traditional female sex role socialization which perpetuates myths that women cannot work together, or prefer to work for a male boss, or are jealous and petty.

Working with Physicians

If as a nursing student you had classes with medical students, this probably has helped you deal with some of the conflicts between nursing and medicine. If not, assertive skills may prove very valuable in developing or holding to an egalitarian collaborative relationship, as opposed to a subservient relationship with physicians. Nursing and medicine bring together different skills and levels of authority as well as competency to give patients professional health care. Therefore, it is important to maintain clear communication and cooperation rather than submit to seductive or patronizing game playing that can obscure the task of patient care and create more ambiguity and distance between nurses and physicians. Interacting as people who have equal interpersonal rights but are trained differently will provide a challenge for both nurses and physicians.

As more nurses obtain master's degrees and doctorates, shared status, prestige, and economic returns will become a reality if assertive stands are taken. This will also change the health care system; women will play more powerful administrative roles. Nurses who hold doctorates may become the hospital administrators or nurses may administrate the entire hospital utilizing not only educational credentials but also management skills learned not only in nursing education but many times learned in keeping a home, juggling meals, housekeeping tasks, and the raising of children. More women will enter medicine and men will feel free to obtain a nursing education. Assertive skills will make this transition possible and nurses' use of self-power to facilitate the process in a caring, humanistic way will be most important.

We must take into account possible negative, emotionally painful risks or consequences that may occur. Often nurses fear that assertive behavior on their part may produce other issues, such as "What if the doctor reports me to the supervisor instead of talking the situation over?" "What if I lose my job by being a patient advocate and holding to what I believe?" "What if my head nurse mistakes my assertion for aggression?" Initial discomfort and worries will occur. However, if you avoid acting assertively, others take advantage and manipulate you for their gain. This is true of people who have power as physicians. Because there are many more long-term benefits and positive outcomes when you behave assertively, you must constantly evaluate your choices. Maintaining respect when you are negotiating with nurses and doctors leaves you with a sense of well-being, feeling in control, and an increased commitment to living.

Avoiding assertive behavior because you fear possible consequences means often that you are resigning yourself to a doormat status and little satisfaction in life. Most physicians appreciate assertive nurses as it becomes obvious someone else is interested and taking responsibility for patient care. This helps physicians discuss and talk over issues. However, physicians who have held the majority of power in the health care system are not going to give it away freely. Nurses who use assertive, competent behavior can obtain more self-power and eventually more power for the nursing profession.

Working with Patients: Teaching Others to Assert Themselves

The patients have a certain responsibility to themselves and to those attending health care professionals to assert their thoughts and feelings regarding not only personal, social, and medical history, but day-to-day health care. If we as nurses have the above expectations regarding patients, we convey the message that patients are an important part of the health care team who have an active involvement in their treatment or hospitalization.

One way to involve the patient more in his care is to encourage him to verbalize thoughts, ideas, and questions. This sounds simple, but the traditional sick role has perpetuated a model of patients sublimating or avoiding feelings and needs, lying passively, and accepting nursing or the medical regime without explanation or concern. In fact, patients forget often that they are people with rights. Consequently, they feel and behave like people inferior to nurses or physicians, mistaking the physical dependence of illness for a lack of worth and importance. Patient conversations often heard in hospital wards validate this inferior status. For example, "It doesn't really matter," or "The doctors are so busy," or "I have a hard time describing how I feel, so I'll be quiet," or "I better not bother anyone as the nurses might get angry and not take care of me."

In our culture somehow being sick means giving up the ability to think or behave independently. As a result, basic fears of not being taken care of are acted out by avoidance of conflict or responsibility to ask for or report changes. However, when a patient is nonassertive oftentimes he doesn't get the proper care since the message does not get communicated to the proper persons. To illustrate, here are some further situations:

Mrs. G. (*Patient*): (*Grimacing*)
Student Nurse: Mrs. G., are you in pain?
Mrs. G.: Oh—yes: They changed my pain medication. Now I get Demerol by mouth and it doesn't do a dang thing for me.
Student Nurse: Have you told the doctor?
Mrs. G.: No, not yet. He's always so busy when he comes around here.

Mr. E. (*patient*): That doctor doesn't tell me anything. One time he says one thing and then later he says something different. I don't think he takes the time to know what he's doing.
R.N.: Have you asked him? Have you asked him about when he plans to put the cast on?
Mr. E.: No—why should he care anyways. He just comes around every day to make sure I'm still here—he has more serious patients than me . . .

In the above two examples, the patients have given up their rights as people to be informed and to make simple requests. This decreases self-esteem and causes increased anxiety.

How have patient's rights been protected? Nurses, organized in the National League for Nursing, pioneered the patients' bill of rights as early as 1959. This document acknowledged that protection of patients' rights was to be the responsibility of the health professionals. In 1973 the American Hospital Association published a patients' bill of rights. This was composed of twelve statements, eight of which were statements concerned with patients' rights to be informed and the remaining four were statements concerned with issues of consideration, respect, privacy, and confidentiality of communication.

In the large group of nurses attending assertion workshops, it was found that nurses believe patients have the following rights:

1. To know health status—given in terms they can understand.
2. To complain—state their needs and feelings.
3. To know what medications are used and what to expect—what the risks are—in all treatments.
4. To refuse medication or treatments—the right to die.
5. To preserve their privacy.
6. To change health providers—as in changing floors.
7. To expect confidentiality.
8. To be treated with respect.
9. To have visitors (not resolved).

Many of these are similar to the other patients' bill of rights.

What has happened to this movement? Although the patients' Bill of Rights (particularly the American Hospital Association's Bill of Rights) was seen as an advancement in allaying patients' fears of uncertainties, many professionals do not recognize or adhere to the document. Their reasons include fears that patients cannot protect themselves, that patients will learn too much, that professionals will not be able to control patients, that their own inadequacies will be revealed. Some patient advocacy programs have been set up but those are different from helping patients to be their own advocates.

Nurses who learn and use assertive skills would be effective patient models in decreasing fears and in terms of speaking out, and this would help patients develop greater feelings of self-worth when ill. Teaching patients to stand up for their rights increases accountability for one's body. In this way, patients can be involved in making decisions about what to have done and what not to have done to their bodies. You, as nurses, can play a large role in teaching and making available the patients' Bill of Rights. Often this may be all that is necessary to reinforce a patient to communicate openly with the nurse or physician. A patient who believes and practices the Bill of Rights immediately becomes a more active agent in his own health care and more accountable to himself. Helping patients progress from patient advocates to helping patients do their own advocacy is a nursing role. This is not to assume nurses will give up the role of patient advocate, but when patients can speak for themselves this helps patients help themselves by lowering their anxiety and brings to them an increased sense of self, all of which complements the healing process.

Urging patients to read the patients' Bill of Rights is often enough to encourage them to communicate openly with you, physicians, and other health professionals. Also a printed form given to each patient would indicate that the hospital stands for patient rights. This would reinforce the idea of patients practicing asserting themselves. However, if a patient is still unassertive, he may need more teaching and "coaching." In the case of Mrs. G., it would have been appropriate for the nurse to say, "Mrs. G., I think it is very important that you tell the doctor that your pain medication is not working since it has been changed. In addition, explaining where the pain is and how it feels is important. Then changing your pain medication to something more effective can be considered. But your physician cannot do this unless you tell him your thoughts and feelings." In addition, the nurse can use role playing with patients who need practice in organizing their thoughts in asking for something or for further information. Nurses modeling assertive behavior also make it possible for patients to learn direct, honest, concise communication. This can occur nurse to nurse, nurse to patient, or nurse to physician. Patients hearing nurses using "I" statements to ask for more information or to challenge comments will more readily learn similar behavior and discover it takes less energy to speak honestly to others. For the patient who feels that the doctor is too busy and doesn't have time to listen to him, it can be emphasized that most doctors are busy, but it is an important part of their work to listen to patients. In addition, it is the patient's right to speak and be heard.

Only with honest and open communication with all health workers can quality health care be provided.

Being a Change Agent

The nursing literature is full of articles on nurses becoming change agents. Assertive training provides the individual nurses with the ability to introduce many changes. Some of the areas in which assertive nurses might function effectively are:

Education: Implement assertion into parts of the curriculum at the undergraduate level so students can begin integrating the skills.

Continuing Education: Present workshops and courses with credit to give additional training and basic training to faculty, administrators, supervisors, public health nurses, and other nurses.

Government: Actively support and lobby for funding and other monies to support nurses. Work to reword nurse practice acts so that independent practitioners have legal support. Work for legislature on health insurance policies so that nurses can receive third-party payments. Become a lobbyist.

Military: Work to reverse sexism in the military. Create other jobs and opportunities for nurse practitioners in the organization.

Recruitment: Publicize advantages of nursing education and encourage nurses who have families to keep in touch with nursing news and consider working on a part-time basis.

Health Teaching: Give health information to patients and consumers. Fight "elitism"—give women information about their bodies so they can make choices. Allow patients to question and challenge present health practices including nursing. Be open to questions on all aspects of life, sex, child-rearing, child abuse, rape, divorce, parenting, marriage, counseling, and encourage patients to discuss when pertinent. Discover how much enjoyment you also get out of this.

Nursing Organizations: Join the ANA and NLN and support their projects and ideas. Actively participate in a committee or run for an office.

Media: Share your accomplishments with the local TV or radio station or newspapers. Encourage the media to sponsor programs that enhance not deprecate the image of nurses.

Consciousness Raising: Encourage nurses to join C.R. groups to enhance and become aware of their attitudes, beliefs, and values regarding women that are constraining to them as professional nurses.

Grants and Articles: Write a grant proposal for an idea to help nursing progress. Find out agencies that are funding and talk to several people. Write and publish articles on issues dealing with nursing.

Community Center Projects: Offer your ideas and knowledge to a community.

Schools: Implement health practices and new job roles for nurses in elementary and secondary schools. Present health-related programs to PTA groups and encourage children to talk about their health potentialities as well as limitations.

REFERENCES

American Hospital Association. *A Patient's Bill of Rights.* Chicago: 1973.

Herman, S. J. "Women, Divorce, and Suicide," *The Journal of Divorce,* 2 (December 1977).

Kelly, L. Y., "The Patients' Right to Know," *Nursing Outlook,* 24, (January 1976): 26–32

The Rights of Patients Public Affairs Pamphlets No. 535 New York: Public Affairs Pamphlets, 381 Park Avenue South.

APPENDIXES

Appendix A: Scripts for Assertive Behavior*

SCRIPTS: REFUSING REQUESTS

1. Male Friend: How about going to dinner tonight?

   Model: No, I have other plans for tonight, but I'd love to go with you another time.

   Male Friend: Great! When will you have free time?

2. Female Colleague: Say, can I borrow your notes from class again? They were really helpful to me on the last exam.

   Model: No, I need them for myself right now. I don't know when exactly I'll be using them, but time is running short till exam time . . .

   Female Colleague: (shrugs) Oh, you're right . . .

3. Nurse: We're selecting a committee to have a neat booth at ANA this year. I've seen you in action and I know you're a good organizer and leader. How about chairing the committee? We could really utilize your talent. All you have to do is be there and help the other nurses to put their ideas together.

   Model: I appreciate your thinking about me, but that amount of work is out of the question for me. I'm having

*The scripts in this Appendix are based on material by Mary Manderino, *Effects of a Group Assertive Training Procedure on Undergraduate Women* (Ann Arbor, Michigan: University Microfilms, 1974); Modified by S. Herman, 1977.

trouble getting through the practitioner program and right now that takes priority over my time.

Nurse: Oh, I didn't realize it was a hassle for you. We'll miss having you help but I understand about the importance of here and now.

4. Co-worker: I've planned to take a long lunch today. Would you mind taking care of my noon meds?

    Assertive Nurse: I'd like to help you out but I've got about all I can handle today. Noontime's a busy time for me.

    Co-worker: Oh, but I just have a few meds. It won't take you long—you're so organized.

    Assertive Nurse: Nancy, I just can't swing it today.

    Co-worker: OK—Guess I'll find someone else.

SCRIPTS: MAKING REQUESTS

1. Classroom situation (*Instructor speaking inaudibly in the background*):

    Model: (*Raises a hand*) I'm having difficulty hearing you back here. Would you please speak a little louder?

    Instructor: Certainly! Can you hear me now?

    Model: That's a little better, but I'm still having trouble.

    Instructor: How's this?

    Model: That's fine. Thanks very much.

2. Model: I loved it the last time you gave me a back rub. Will you give me another one now?

    Boyfriend: Sure! I enjoy it too.

3. Model: Dr. Blank, I can't seem to understand that formula you went over in class today. I know you went over it a number of times, but I can't get it through my head.

    Instructor: Suppose you see the T.A.? His job is to help clarify the lectures.

    Model: I went to see him and he wasn't available—I'd really

like to understand this as soon as possible. It seems crucial to understanding the rest of the chapter.

Instructor: Get out your notebook. . . . Now, where are you having difficulty?

4. Restaurant situation:

Waiter: How is everything with you folks?

Model: Not so good. I ordered a medium rare steak and this is quite overdone. I'd appreciate it if you would take this back to the kitchen and have another one fixed for me.

Waiter: *(Peers at steak)* You've already cut into it! It *has* a medium rare sticker on it.

Model: But it is *not* medium rare. Please take it back for me.

Waiter: *(Abruptly snatches the plate up and grumbles as he leaves)* The chef will have a fit.

5. Assertive Nurse: I've been assigned to do an ice lavage—I'm not at all sure of how to do this. Would you mind running through the procedure with me?

Co-worker: I'd be happy to. I wish more people would check out procedures they're unsure of.

SCRIPTS: ASKING FOR A CHANGE IN BEHAVIOR

Structured Scripts

1. Model: Lately, you have been doing a lot of noisy things while I'm studying—like turning up the stereo and dancing around—having long conversations on the phone. When you do these things I have trouble concentrating. I get to feeling up tight and then angry with you. I'd like for you to be a little quieter while I'm at my desk. We've been roommates for a year now and I've very much enjoyed sharing this room together. I just don't want to build up resentments toward you. I don't want anything to get in the way of our friendship.

Roomate: I'm glad you told me about that. I'll sure remember to be quiet next time. Noise doesn't bother me when I study, so I assumed it couldn't bother you either.

2. Model: Well, this is how I feel about the Equal Rights Amendment.

    Boyfriend: (*Interrupts her*) Hey, did you hear about Billie Jean King?

    Model: You just interrupted me. You have been doing that a lot lately. When you do that, I feel very unimportant—insignificant—sort of put down. When I say things to you, I'd like for you to hear me out—let me finish.

    Boyfriend: I didn't know I was doing that. I don't mean to put you down. Would you let me know the next time it happens?

    Model: Yes, I'll do that. That sounds like a way for us to have a better relationship.

3. Model: You have not been helping me keep this room very neat. I don't like to live in a mess—yet I resent being the only one to straighten things out. The more I pick up after you, the angrier I get. I'd like for you to at least make your bed every day and pick up after yourself.

    Roommate: Look! I'm busy! I don't have time to be doing a lot of housekeeping. God, you're compulsive!

    Model: Does that mean you're not going to change?

    Roommate: I don't mind living the way I do. Why don't you relax a little? Some day you'll realize that having a tidy little room is *not* the most important thing in the world.

    Model: Well, you happen to be very important to me. I like having you as a roommate and as a good friend, but this cleaning thing is getting in my way. I'd like for us to work it out some way.

    Roommate: Our relationship is important to me, too, so let's talk it over and see what we can do.

4. Model: When you tell me you are going to come over to see me and don't show up, I feel hurt—left hanging. Then I feel

angry because I've waited around for you all night. I want
for you to either follow through with what you said you'd do
or give me a call to let me know you changed your mind. I
want for our relationship to continue, but this is really
getting in my way.

Boyfriend: Sometimes I forget—I'm just so busy. I don't
mean to hurt you. Give a guy a break, will you?

Model: This has happened *four* or *five* times the last month.
I want to let you know that if you don't show up or call
within a reasonable length of time—like a half hour, I will
have other plans.

Boyfriend: Okay, okay. I get the message. I'll remember
next time.

5. Model: Dad, there's something that's bugging me about
    you, and I want to talk to you about it.

    Father: So, what's bothering you about me?

    Model: Lately, you have been very critical of the guys I have
    been going out with. Every time I introduce you to a guy,
    you point out all the things you don't like about him. You tell
    me in essence that he's not good enough for me. When you
    do that, I feel put down . . . like a child who can't make a
    decision.

    Father: Now, wait a minute, honey. . . . I just want you to
    have the very best.

    Model: I know you do, and I appreciate that very much.
    What I'm saying is that I want to make my own judgments
    and decisions about the fellows I go out with. I'd like for you
    not to give your opinions so that I can make my mind up
    independently.

    Father: I just can't stand by and let you go out with those
    long-haired weirdos. You still need my advice . . . whether
    you like it or not.

    Model: There are times, Dad, when I want your advice. The
    point is with regard to whom I do or do not date . . . I want to
    take only my own advice . . . make my own mistakes.

Father: Well, all I can say is you give yourself pretty poor advice. You're still going out with that Kramer bum. Tell me, what's he got going for him. Lives off his parents' money still.

Model: Dad, you're doing what I asked you not to do. If you continue to criticize the way you have been doing, I simply will not bring my boyfriends here. I want for them to know you and you them . . . that's important to me. But it is also important that I learn to make my own decisions about people.

Father: (*Shrugs—throws up his hands*) What can I say?

6. Head Nurse: Dr. King I need to speak with you for a moment.

Doctor: Well, make it fast. I'm in a hurry.

Head Nurse: I would very much appreciate it if you would come an hour earlier for rounds. As it is now, you've been coming in at our very busiest time and you've gotten angry when we haven't been able to work with you immediately.

Doctor: Well, I'm a busy man! I don't like to be kept waiting.

Head Nurse: Yes. That's just it. We'd like not to keep you waiting. I feel very frustrated when you come at our very busy time. If you could come about an hour earlier, it would be a perfect time for us and you won't have to be waiting around.

Doctor: Okay—I'll take another look at my schedule.

GIVING A COMPLIMENT

Nurse: I just saw you bathing Mrs. Anderson and I couldn't help but notice how you were not only taking care of her physical needs, but were also so supportive of her emotionally. It was obvious by the way you listened and responded to her that you really care about her.

Aide: It feels good to hear that. I did feel that I was being helpful to Mrs. Anderson.

COPING WITH UNCLEAR CRITICISM

Co-worker: Boy, you sure are scattered sometimes.

Assertive Nurse: I'm not sure what you mean. How am I scattered?

Co-worker: Well you're so disorganized!

Assertive Nurse: Could you give me an example of what you mean?

Co-worker: Well, your lab requests are always late.

Assertive Nurse: What else about my behavior is disorganized?

Co-worker: Well, nothing else really. But it does make me mad when I have to make special trips for lab procedures.

Assertive Nurse: I understand what you're saying now. I had no idea I was creating a problem for you. Thanks for letting me know.

COPING WITH APPROPRIATE CRITICISM

Head Nurse: You sure blew it. Mr. Jones' veins are shot! After one attempt with such fragile veins you absolutely should notify the I.V. team.

Assertive Nurse: You're right. I realized too late that I needed help. I sure won't let this happen again!

EXAMPLES OF INDIRECT AGGRESSIVE BEHAVIOR OR MANIPULATION

Flattery:	How's my efficient nurse? By the way, would you run this down to the lab.
	or
	How's the floor tonight? It amazes me how you always have everything under control. Okay, hand me my charts, please.
Ridicule:	I thought nurses were tough, not emotional.

You're slipping Miss Smith.

or

Just throw it on the floor, the nurses don't have anything to do.

Psychoanalyzing: You've been taking a course in assertion, I can tell. You got it all together now? I'll have to watch out for you.

Helplessness: I can't get Mrs. X. to stop complaining of pain. Would you do something?

Guilt Induction: All right, don't come in this weekend—we can make it without you. Oh, we'll manage . . . somehow. Don't worry about a thing, enjoy your time off.

or

You certainly sound hostile. You wouldn't think of expressing that hostility during the committee meeting would you?

Generalizing: You always sound tired; you are always late; you always know all the answers. (*Ask for specifics.*)

Seduction: Start working for me at this level of salary and rotating shifts and when we get more help you can have a place on days.

Vagueness: Everything is quiet tonight, take my word for it. You only have to watch Mr. Smith.

Illness: You give me a headache. You're really off your rocker.

No Fight: Person maintains silence and seems to agree but doesn't.

Appendix B: Teaching Nurses Assertive Behavior: Special Considerations

This book is written as a self-help guide for nurses learning assertiveness. It is not to be used to train assertive trainers. For specifics for those nurses interested in teaching assertion, the author refers you to Appendix C, which gives a statement of "Principles for Ethical Practice of Assertive Behavior Training." In teaching nurses several other considerations are important.

QUALIFICATIONS OF THE TRAINER

Nurses who have an advanced graduate degree in the area of psychiatric-mental health nursing skills or other counseling advanced degrees have the basic requirements for learning a behavior approach to assertion training. It is highly recommended that nurses comply with "Principles for Ethical Practice of Assertive Behavior Training." Equally important, the nurse trainer should be fully acquainted not only with nursing but the health care system so that she can matter-of-factly present nursing socialization conflicts and effectively model alternative assertive behavior. A nurse who can honestly speak her views in front of a group of nurses without fear or hesitation (1) of having the approval of every nurse listening, (2) that she will be seen as aggressive, (3) that she perfectly models assertive behavior, will be an effective assertive trainer for nurses. This assertive role model is necessary as it provides permission for other nurses to stand up and speak to issues in which they believe. Female nurse trainers are highly recommended.

By observing an assertive role model nurses can more easily confront the female sex role conditioning compounded by the nursing socialization process, which has perpetuated blind obedience rather than a questioning or challenging approach in work and educational settings. Female nurses who have been socialized to exist for others and to consider everyone else's needs first will best learn from female assertive role models who use a problem-solving approach to teach and reinforce individual rights.

Male trainers, especially if they are not nurses, often reinforce the female conditional training and belief system of nurses (see Chapter 7). This is true particularly in regard to nurses' beliefs regarding physicians. Male trainers symbolically represent the physicians and this only impedes assertive training and reinforces traditional learning (Herman, 1977; Adams, 1977). This dynamic has been obvious in a number of workshops for nurses taught by males. Instead of being direct in the sessions with one another nurses began to be more indirect (Herman, 1977).

Equally important as the nurses' academic credentials are her personal qualities of honesty, openness, and authenticity as an individual (Rogers, 1961). Being emotionally honest in a communication interaction rather than withdrawing, ordering, or manipulating the other person brings increased self-respect to the nurse and to the other person. This happens when two people are not competing with each other to win an interaction but are sharing honest thoughts and feelings in an egalitarian situation about issues. Since nurses have too often been manipulated, a trainer modeling authenticity will promote trust and permission for nurses to respond with emotional honesty. This provides for flexible compromise and negotiations.

USING BEHAVIOR THERAPY PRINCIPLES TO TEACH ASSERTIVENESS

Teaching or learning assertiveness using a behavior therapy

approach means practicing new behavior, unlearning old behavior, and building positive belief systems before attitudes are changed. This approach is different from most methods of the teaching-learning process in nursing. In nursing education, it is often assumed that attitudes must be changed before behavior. While theorists have debated whether it is important to first change attitudes or behavior, it is evident from studies mentioned in this book and from personal research that changing behavior can be an effective short-term intervention. For example, following use of an assertive response, a change may be noticed in how others respond to you. Most often this is positive feedback, which is a satisfying reinforcement for a formerly self-denying nonassertive nurse. When this occurs, as it often does after the first sessions, attitudes toward the self begin to change significantly to correspond with the new behavior. Awareness occurs that "I am responsible for the positive response in myself and from others." This increases self-esteem and lowers anxiety. Nurses, after a two-hour session, often make comments like, "I went home and directly shared some feelings with my husband. He liked it and said he wished I would do that often", or "I said 'no' to a request without a smile on my face and my adolescent daughter not only accepted the 'no' but did not try and manipulate me as she usually does."

FORMATS IN WHICH TO TEACH ASSERTION

Offering assertion training in a workshop format is an effective manner in which to present the material to nurses. In a workshop format more freedom to learn concepts can be permitted without the students being graded. It provides a more informal setting in which it can be fun to learn.

This method provides a way nurses can learn assertion in small or large groups while at the same time building on the participating nurses' own competence and expertise to help themselves and other nurses. Learning assertion and helping others can enable nurses to increase positive feelings about one another. For too long nurses have been pitted against each other, set up to compete for who could be the best nurse, or who could gain the doctor's approval or even be the favorite. By teaching assertion in which the interdependence of the learners is increased, when all role playing is done in triads, for example, opportunities to give positive and valid feedback are provided. Nurses helping each other learn from each other, rather than looking to traditional authority figures who model how one ought to be. The workshop format of teaching assertion encourages nurses to look at themselves, challenge the assumptions that others know what's best for them, begin to make personal conscious choices of what to say, when and where, and to actively practice new behavior.

Assertion training can also be taught as a course with credit within the graduate nursing curriculum (Manderino, 1976) or as a three-credit undergraduate course as was given nursing students in the Walter Reed Institute for Nurses program in Washington, D.C. Courses provide material in more depth than the workshop format and the nature of role playing can help build in an ongoing authentic group support system. Students can contract for grades if they can't be given as pass/fail. Both undergraduate and graduate students seem to be eager to present problems and role play different alternatives.

Integrating assertive concepts into a nursing curriculum is another alternative. Nursing students at The Johns Hopkins University were taught beginning assertion in an interpersonal course, intermediate assertion skills in the psychiatric-nursing course, and then encouraged to attend one of the biannual assertive training workshops held at the University. Students were encouraged to collect examples and write papers on applying assertiveness, integrating interpersonal rights, and nursing. This can be expanded in other ways in the future.

These considerations are not only special to teaching assertiveness to nurses but facilitate the entire learning spectrum of the nurse. Such considerations seemed to help nurses experience less resistance to behavioral rehearsal of assertive behavior and to participate more readily in evaluating self and others with emotionally valid feedback.

REFERENCES

Adams, M. Assertiveness and Management Training for Nurses. Unpublished research. Academy of Health Sciences, Behavioral Science Division, Fort Sam Houston, Texas, 1976.

Herman, S.J. "Stereotypic Beliefs of Nurses." Unpublished paper presented at The Johns Hopkins University Assertion Training Workshop, February 1977.

Mandarino, M.A. "Comments on Teaching Nurses Assertiveness," *Journal of Continuing Education of Nurses*, (March-April 1976): 80-81.

Rogers, C.R. *On Becoming a Person*. Massachusetts: Houghton-Mifflin Company, 1961.

Appendix C: A Statement of "Principles for Ethical Practice of Assertive Behavior Training"*

With the increasing popularity of assertive behavior training, a quality of "faddishness" has become evident, and there are frequent reports of ethically irresponsible practices (and practitioners). We hear of trainers who, for example, do not adequately differentiate assertion and aggression. Others have failed to advocate proper ethical responsibility and caution to clients—e.g., failed to alert them to and/or prepare them for the possibility of retaliation or other highly negative reactions from others.

The following statement of "Principles for Ethical Practice of Assertive Behavior Training" is the work of the professional psychologists and educators listed below, who are actively engaged in the practice of facilitating assertive behavior (also referred to as "assertive therapy," "social skills training," "personal effectiveness training," and "AT"). We don't intend by this statement to discourage untrained individuals from becoming more assertive on their own, and we don't advocate that one must have extensive credentials in order to be of help to friends and relatives. Rather, these principles are offered to help foster responsible and ethical teaching and practice by human services professionals. Others who wish to enhance their own assertiveness or that of associates are encouraged to do so, with

*From *Assert: The Newsletter of Assertive Behavior.* Copyright © 1976, Impact Publishers, Inc., San Luis Obispo, California, 93406. Reprinted by permission.

awareness of their own limitations, and of the importance of seeking help from a qualified therapist/trainer when necessary.

We hereby declare support for and adherence to the statement of principles, and invite responsible professionals in our own and other fields who use these techniques to join us in advocating and practicing these principles.

Robert E. Alberti, Ph.D.
Counseling Psychologist & Professor
California Polytechnic State University
San Luis Obispo, CA

Michael L. Emmons, Ph.D.
Counseling Psychologist & Professor
California Polytechnic State University
San Luis Obispo, CA

Iris G. Fodor, Ph.D.
Associate Professor, Educational Psychology
New York University, Washington Square
New York, NY

John Galassi, Ph.D.
School of Education
University of North Carolina
Chapel Hill, NC

Merna D. Galassi, Ed.D.
Meredith College
Raleigh, NC

Lynne Garnett, Ph.D.
Counseling Psychologist
University of California
Los Angeles, CA

Patricia Jakubowski, Ed.D.
Associate Professor, Behavior Studies
University of Missouri
St. Louis, MO

Janet L. Wolfe, Ph.D.
Director of Clinical Services
Institute for Advanced Study in Rational Psychotherapy
New York, NY

                                                    May 1, 1976

1. Definition of Assertive Behavior

For purposes of these principles and the ethical framework expressed herein, we define assertive behavior as that complex of behaviors, emitted by a person in an interpersonal context, which express that person's feelings, attitudes, wishes, opinions or rights directly, firmly, and honestly, while respecting the feelings, attitudes, wishes, opinions and rights of the other person(s). Such behavior may include the expression of such emotions as anger, fear, caring, hope, joy, despair, indignance, embarrassment, but in any event is expressed in a manner which does not violate the rights of others. Assertive behavior is differentiated from aggressive behavior which, while expressive of one person's feelings, attitudes, wishes, opinions or rights, does not respect those characteristics in others.

While this definition is intended to be comprehensive, it is recognized that any adequate definition of assertive behavior must consider several dimensions:

A.   Intent: behavior classified as assertive is not intended by its author to be hurtful of others.

B.   Behavior: behavior classified as assertive would be evaluated by an "objective observer" as itself honest, direct, expressive and non-destructive of others.

C.   Effects: behavior classified as assertive has the effect upon the receiver of a direct and non-destructive message, by which a "reasonable person" would not be hurt.

D.   Socio-cultural Context: behavior classified as assertive is appropriate to the environment and culture in which it is exhibited, and may not be considered "assertive" in a different socio-cultural environment.

2. Client Self-Determination

These principles recognize and affirm the inherent dignity

and the equal and inalienable rights of all members of the human family, as proclaimed in the "Universal Declaration of Human Rights" endorsed by the General Assembly of the United Nations.

Pursuant to the precepts of the Declaration, each client (trainee, patient) who seeks assertive behavior training shall be treated as a person of value, with all of the freedoms and rights expressed in the Declaration. No procedure shall be utilized in the name of assertive behavior training which would violate those freedoms or rights.

Informed client self-determination shall guide all such interventions:

A. the client shall be fully informed in advance of all procedures to be utilized;
B. the client shall have the freedom to choose to participate or not at any point in the intervention;
C. the client who is institutionalized shall be similarly treated with respect and without coercion, insofar as is possible within the institutional environment;
D. the client shall be provided with explicit definitions of assertiveness and assertive training;
E. the client shall be fully informed as to the education, training, experience or other qualifications of the assertive trainer(s);
F. the client shall be informed as to the goals and potential outcomes of assertive training, including potentially high levels of anxiety, and possible negative reactions from others;
G. the client shall be fully informed as to the responsibility of the assertion trainer(s) and the client(s);
H. the client shall be informed as to the ethics and employment of confidentiality guidelines as they pertain to various assertive training settings (e.g., clinical vs. non-clinical).

3. Qualifications of Facilitators

Assertive behavior training is essentially a therapeutic procedure, although frequently practiced in a variety of settings by professionals not otherwise engaged in rendering a "psychological" service. Persons in any professional role who engage in helping others to change their behavior, attitudes, and interpersonal relationships must understand human behavior at a level commensurate with the level of their interventions.

3.1 *General Qualifications*

We support the following minimum, general qualifications for facilitators at all levels of intervention (including "trainers in training"—preservice or inservice—who are preparing for professional service in a recognized human services field, and who may be conducting assertive behavior training under supervision as part of a research project or practicum):

A.   Fundamental understanding of the principles of learning and behavior (equivalent to completion of a rigorous undergraduate level course in learning theory);

B.   Fundamental understanding of anxiety and its effects upon behavior (equivalent to completion of a rigorous undergraduate level course in abnormal psychology);

C.   Knowledge of the limitations, contraindications and potential dangers of assertive behavior training; familiarity with theory and research in the area.

D.   Satisfactory evidence of competent performance as a facilitator, as observed by a qualified trainer, is strongly recommended for all professionals, particularly for those who do not possess a doctorate or an equivalent level of training. Such evidence would most ideally be supported by:

1)   participation in at least ten (10) hours of assertive behavior training as a client (trainee, patient); and

2)   participation in at least ten (10) hours of assertive behavior training as a facilitator under supervision.

3.2 *Specific Qualifications*

The following additional qualifications are considered to be the minimum expected for facilitators at the indicated levels of intervention:

A.   Assertive behavior training, including non-clinical workshops, groups, and individual client training aimed at teaching assertive skills to those persons who require only encouragement and specific skill training, and in whom no serious emotional deficiency or pathology is evident.

1) For trainers in programs conducted under the sponsorship of a recognized human services agency, school, governmental or corporate entity, church, or community organization:

   a) An advanced degree in a recognized field of human services (e.g., psychology, counseling, social work, medicine, public health, nursing, education, human development, theology/divinity), including at least one term of field experience in a human services agency supervised by a qualified trainer; or

   b) certification as a minister, public school teacher, social worker, physician, counselor, nurse, or clinical, counseling, educational, or school psychologist, or similar human services professional, as recognized by the state wherein employed or by the recognized state or national professional society in the indicated discipline; or

   c) one year of paid counseling experience in a recognized human services agency, supervised by a qualified trainer; or

   d) qualification under items 3.2B or 3.2C below.

2) For trainers in programs including interventions at the level defined in this item (3.2A), but without agency/organization sponsorship:

   a) An advanced degree in a recognized field of human services (e.g., psychology, counseling, social work, medicine, public health, nursing, education, human development, theology/divinity) including at least one term of field experience in a human services agency supervised by a qualified trainer; and

   b) certification as a minister, social worker, physician, counselor, nurse, or clinical, counseling, educational, or school psychologist, or similar human services professional, as recognized by

the state wherein employed or by the recognized
state or national professional society in the indicated discipline; or

c) qualification under items 3.2B or 3.2C below.

B. Assertive behavior therapy, including clinical interventions designed to assist persons who are severely inhibited by anxiety, or who are significantly deficient in social
skills, or who are controlled by aggression, or who
evidence pathology, or for whom other therapeutic procedures are indicated:

1) For therapists in programs conducted under the
sponsorship of a recognized human services agency,
school, governmental or corporate entity, church, or
community organization:

a) An advanced degree in a recognized field of
human services (e.g., psychology, counseling,
social work, medicine, public health, nursing,
education, human development, theology/divin-
ity) including at least one term of field experience in a human services agency supervised by
a qualified trainer; or

b) certification as a minister, social worker, physician, counselor, nurse, or clinical, counseling,
educational, or school psychologist, as recognized by the state wherein employed or by the
recognized state or national professional society
in the individual discipline; or

c) qualification under item 3.2C below.

2) For therapists employing interventions at the level
defined in this item (3.2B), but without agency/or-
ganization sponsorship:

a) An advanced degree in a recognized field of
human services (e.g., psychology, counseling,
social work, medicine, public health, nursing,
education, human development, theology/divin-
ity) including at least one term of field experience in a human services agency supervised by
a qualified trainer; and

   b) certification as minister, social worker, physician, counselor, nurse, or clinical, counseling, educational, or school psychologist, as recognized by the state wherein employed or by the recognized state or national professional society in the indicated discipline; and

   c) at least one year of paid professional experience in a recognized human services agency, supervised by a qualified trainer; or

   d) qualification under item 3.2C below.

C. Training of trainers, including preparation of other professionals to offer assertive behavior training/therapy to clients, in school, agency, organization, or individual settings:

  1) A doctoral degree in a recognized field of human services (e.g., psychology, counseling, social work, medicine, public health, nursing, education, human development, theology/divinity) including at least one term of field experience in a human services agency supervised by a qualified trainer; and

  2) certification as a minister, social worker, physician, counselor, nurse, or clinical, counseling, educational, or school psychologist, as recognized by the state wherein employed, or by the recognized state or national professional society in the indicated discipline; and

  3) at least one year of paid professional experience in a recognized human services agency, supervised by a qualified trainer; and

  4) advanced study in assertive behavior training/therapy, including at least two of the following:

   a) At least thirty (30) hours of facilitation with clients;

   b) participation in at least two different workshops at professional meetings or professional training institutes;

   c) contribution to the professional literature in the field.

3.3 We recognize that counselors and psychologists are not certified by each state. In states wherein no such certification is provided, unless contrary to local statute, we acknowledge the legitimacy of professionals who: A) are otherwise qualified under the provisions of items 3.1 and 3.2; and B) would be eligible for certification as a counselor or psychologist in another state.

3.4 We do not consider that participation in one or two workshops on assertive behavior, even though conducted by a professional with an advanced degree, is adequate qualification to offer assertive behavior training to others, unless the additional qualifications of items 3.1 and 3.2 are also met.

3.5 These qualifications are presented as standards for professional facilitators of assertive behavior. No "certification" or "qualifying" agency is hereby proposed. Rather, it is incumbent upon each professional to evaluate himself/herself as a trainer/therapist according to these standards, and to make explicit to clients the adequacy of his/her qualifications as a facilitator.

4. Ethical Behavior of Facilitators

Since the encouragement and facilitation of assertive behavior is essentially a therapeutic procedure, the ethical standards most applicable to the practice of assertive behavior training are those of psychologists. We recognize that many persons who practice some form of assertive behavior training are not otherwise engaged in rendering a "psychological" service (i.e., teachers, personnel/training directors). To all we support the statement of "Ethical Standards for Psychologists" as adopted by the American Psychological Association as the standard of ethical behavior by which assertive behavior training shall be conducted.

We recognize that the methodology employed in assertive behavior training may include a wide range of procedures, some of which are of unproven value. It is the responsibility of facilitators to inform clients of any experimental procedures. Under no circumstances should the facilitator "guarantee" a specific outcome from an intervention.

5. Appropriateness of Assertive Behavior Training Interventions

Assertive behavior training, as any intervention oriented toward helping people change, may be applied under a wide range of conditions, yet its appropriateness must be evaluated in each individual case. The responsible selection of assertive behavior training for a particular intervention must include attention to at least the following dimensions:

A. Client: The personal characteristics of the client in question (age, sex, ethnicity, institutionalization, capacity for informed choice, physical and psychological functionality).

B. Problem/Goals: The purpose for which professional help has been sought or recommended (job skills, severe inhibition, anxiety reduction, overcome aggression).

C. Facilitator: The personal and professional qualifications of the facilitator in question (age, sex, ethnicity, skills, understanding, ethics—see also Principles 3 and 4 above).

D. Setting: The characteristics of the setting in which the intervention is conducted (home, school, business, agency, clinic, hospital, prison). Is the client free to choose? Is the facilitator's effectiveness systematically evaluated?

E. Time/Duration: The duration of the intervention. Does the time involved represent a brief word of encouragement, a formal training workshop, an intensive and long-term therapeutic effort?

F. Method: The nature of the intervention. Is it a "packaged" procedure or tailored to client needs? Is training based on sound principles of learning and behavior? Is there clear differentiation of aggressiveness, assertiveness and other concepts? Are definitions, techniques, procedures and purposes clarified? Is care taken to encourage small, successful steps and to minimize punishing consequences? Are any suggested "homework assignments" presented with adequate supervision, responsibility, and sensitivity to the effect upon significant others of the client's behavior change efforts? Are clients informed that assertiveness "doesn't always work?"

G.   Outcome: Are there follow-up procedures, either by self-report or other post-test procedures?

6. Social Responsibility

Assertive behavior training shall be conducted within the law. Trainers and clients are encouraged to work assertively to change those laws which they consider need to be changed, and to modify the social system in ways they believe appropriate—in particular to extend the boundaries of human rights. Toward these ends, trainers are encouraged to facilitate responsible change skills via assertive behavior training. All those who practice, teach, or do research on assertive behavior are urged to advocate caution and ethical responsibility in application of the technique, in accordance with these Principles.

INDEX